DATA-DRIVEN HEALTHCARE IMPROVEMENT:

A Recipe for Provider Excellence

Henry Johnson, MD, MPH
Dustin J. Richardson
NoraZoë Woolridge, MBA, M.Ed

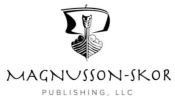

MAGNUSSON-SKOR
PUBLISHING, LLC

Denver

Published by

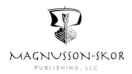

Magnusson-Skor Publishing
4600 S. Ulster Street, Suite 1050
Denver, CO 80237

Library of Congress Cataloging-in-Publication Data

Johnson, Henry C. L., Jr
Richardson, Dustin J.
Woolridge, NoraZoë

Data-Driven Healthcare Improvement: A Recipe for Provider Excellence.
p. cm.
Includes biographical references.
ISBN 978-0-9842051-3-4
1. Physician Profiling 2. Healthcare Improvement 3. Accreditation I. Title

First Edition

DISCLAIMER

Although the authors and publisher have made every effort to ensure that the information in this book is correct at press time, the authors and publisher do not assume and hereby disclaim any liability to any party for any loss, damage, or disruption caused by errors or omissions, whether such errors or omissions result from negligence, accident, or any other cause.

This book is presented solely for informational, experiential, and educational purposes. The authors and publisher are not offering it as legal, medical, operational, or other professional services advice. While best efforts have been used in preparing this book, the authors and publisher make no representations or warranties of any kind and assume no liabilities of any kind with respect to the accuracy or completeness of the contents and specifically disclaim any implied warranties of merchantability or fitness of use for a particular purpose.

Neither the authors nor the publisher shall be held liable or responsible to any person or entity with respect to any loss or incidental or consequential damages caused, or alleged to have been caused, directly or indirectly, by the information contained herein. No warranty may be created or extended by sales representatives or written sales materials.

Every organization is different and the advice and strategies contained herein may not be suitable for your situation, business, medical group, hospital, or practice. You should seek the services of a competent professional before making changes to Medical Staff policies, procedures, actions, or activities. References and citations are included to the best of our abilities at the time of writing.

In regard to accreditation standards, the authors have done their best to represent them, as we understand them at the time of publication, providing references that are current as of the publication date. Standards are open to interpretation and change over time. For final interpretation of standards consult with your accrediting agency.

Table of Contents

For Dr. Christopher J. Heller, co-founder of Midas+.

A skilled and compassionate surgeon, Dr. Heller enjoyed limitless intellectual curiosity and a vision of better and safer patient care through analysis of data.

You could not have had a better physician or a better friend.

We would like to start by thanking Dr. Christopher Heller, for his lifelong commitment to caring for children and adults, as well as his unfaltering work to improve clinical care through performance improvement at all levels within health care organizations. His work on provider profiling has created the foundation for this volume.

We recognize all our colleagues at Midas+ for their dedication to our clients and their work over the years to help each client perform a little better each day. Likewise, we acknowledge many of our colleagues, who, through their work with clients, have built on the foundation of provider-centric metrics. We know how hard they work, and we appreciate their contributions.

We would like to thank all our clients with whom we have had the privilege of working over the years. Their focus on all areas of performance improvement has informed the content of this book, and helps guide the trajectory of progress in this discipline. We learn from them every day.

Special appreciation goes to our colleagues who have taken the time to review early drafts of this manuscript, providing suggestions, support, and guidance. You have been our compass.

Special thanks to Dr. Mark Montoney and Nina Bush at Tenet Healthcare, who were willing to read an early draft and provide suggestions that have made this volume better. And thanks to Dr. Richard Dutton, Executive Director of the Anesthesia Quality Institute, for his document review and insights on the text of the Chapter 4 section on Anesthesia. His informed perspective was invaluable.

Finally, thanks to all our families and friends for supporting us in so many ways as we pursued this manuscript. Anyone who has written a book can attest to the time demands it imposes, especially as it nears completion.

One thing is constant in healthcare: change. People's needs change. Research findings change. Treatments change. Medications change. Technologies change. Government regulations change. Societies change. This means that the models of care must constantly adapt to strike the balance between consistent, repeatable, high-quality, cost-effective care and the ever-changing needs, knowledge, and abilities to deliver this care. Ultimately, providers have a tremendous responsibility to always strive for the next level of excellence in delivering care while compassionately educating and inspiring patients to become actively involved in their own personal health.

We at Midas+ Solutions, a Xerox Company, have learned there are important steps within change. A good first step is to acknowledge that to progress, to move forward, change is required. As George Bernard Shaw said, "Progress is impossible without change, and those who cannot change their minds cannot change anything."

Another key step we can agree upon is that we must be willing to change and must take personal ownership in change. In the words of Jim Rohn, "You must take personal responsibility. You cannot change the circumstances, the seasons, or the wind, but you can change yourself. That is something you have charge of."

Finally, we must be willing to engage in continuous process improvement and understand that change is a journey, not an event. Transparency is an essential part of continuous quality improvement. I believe Winston Churchill captured it well when he stated, "To improve is to change; to be perfect is to change often." To change often, we must be able to dependably and frequently see and understand our results.

There is no perfect healthcare model in the world today, but there are tremendous efforts and new findings on a daily basis. The more we engage in transparent and consistent review of our processes and outcomes in a meaningful and comparative way, the better we are able to work together on this journey to discover where the opportunities exist for improvement and to measure how our efforts impact our results.

At Midas+, during our more than 27 years in the healthcare arena, we have come to truly embrace the reality of constant change. Our commitment to prioritizing the best ways to impact care outcomes and the most effective means of delivering solutions and services aligns us with healthcare organizations across the country that are likewise committed to achieving their goals with their patients, their medical staffs, and their communities.

This book provides a wonderful recipe. Laying the foundation for a pragmatic, repeatable, and dependable way to evaluate the providers of healthcare on this journey is essential. We understand how vital it is to track the performance of providers for regulatory organizations. This need is detailed thoroughly in this book, resulting in a shared comprehension, allowing us to be 'on the same page', and enabling an increased ability to share insights and grow together. What may be even more important, however, is how the recipe in this book supports the medical staff itself in its quest to change, to develop, and to grow.

We at Midas+ are pleased to have supported the development of this book and to have contributed thought leadership via the sharing of our colleagues and the nearly 30 years of knowledge on this topic that spans more than 2,000 of our healthcare partners. We hope that this book offers you pragmatic steps, guidance, and best practices from research across the industry.

Justin W. Lanning
SVP, Managing Director
Midas+ Solutions, a Xerox Company

This book is the result of many years of work on building provider profiles along with our clients at Midas+, a Xerox Company, in Tucson, Arizona. It began with the work of one of the company's co-founders, Dr. Christopher J. Heller, to whom this volume is dedicated.

As Dr. Heller and one of us, Dr. Johnson, began to present via webinar and at the company's annual symposium, we discovered great benefit associated with comparing the process of designing and building profiles to cooking a meal. The alignment was clear; necessary elements included understanding who was coming to dinner (the physicians and other practitioners); knowing what they wanted to eat to build the menu (designing the final profile or scorecard); shopping for the right ingredients at the right price (getting the data within a budget); being sure that everything was fresh (checking the data for Validity, Accuracy, and Reliability); building the profiles (cooking); and, finally, the meal's presentation (implementation and adoption).

We have decided to continue this analogy throughout this volume in the form of call-outs interspersed at appropriate locations within the chapters. This allows the reader to get an occasional chuckle, and provides a familiar framework to structure otherwise new ideas and workflow. Additional call-outs provide content related to various topics.

Let us pause at the outset, for a word about terminology. Although we started building *physician profiles* with our clients, we were really building *profiles, scorecards*, or *reports on the clinical performance of licensed independent practitioners*, most of whom happened to be physicians – MDs or DOs. Because of this broader scope, and in our hopes to write inclusively, we have decided to use the following terminology in this volume.

We have borrowed the phrase *Professional Practice* from The Joint Commission's term *Ongoing Professional Practice Evaluation*, to refer to what licensed independent practitioners do. The scorecard or report of his or her own performance that each practitioner reviews is a *Professional Practice Profile*. When these profiles are reviewed by professional leadership, it is a *Professional Practice Evaluation*.

Over the years, we have learned coming to agreement on terminology can be a challenge; however, as authors, we offer the following vendor-neutral terms. In regard to the profiles themselves, some Medical Staffs prefer the term *Scorecard*, others prefer *Care Reports*, and still others are content with *Profiles*. The choice is yours; you do not have to use our terminology, but we do need to be clear and consistent as we write this volume. We will therefore attempt to use the term *Profile* when referring to the evaluative measures included for a provider to view to assess his or her own performance. We will likewise use the term *Profile* and the verb *Profiling* to describe a specialty or a group's collective performance metrics.

For our purposes, we understand *Professionals* to be medical practitioners who are being evaluated through the Medical Staff Office, not by your hospital's human resources department. These individuals include nurse practitioners and physician assistants, in addition to licensed physicians with MD or DO degrees.

So get ready, here it comes: how to design and build *Professional Practice Profiles* to ensure data-driven healthcare improvement.

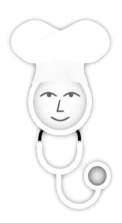

Introduction

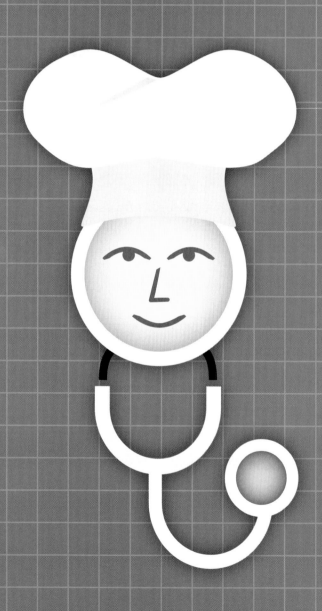

Menus and Ingredients

The process of creating and delivering provider profiles is not too different from planning, preparing, cooking, and serving a meal. In both cases, we need to know who is coming to dinner, or identify our customers/consumers first. Then, we need to understand what they want or need to eat so we can plan the menu in advance.

Determining the menu can be tricky. The Joint Commission has outlined a minimum number of items to be served via profiles, and recommends how they should be presented, but the Medical Staff members themselves are picky eaters. We must meet their needs, since this meal is really for them. Face it: they are your most important diners and customers. So, while you prepare the meal for them, also be sure that your accrediting organization is happy with your offering.

As you plan the menu, start small and build over time. Many of us wish we could be gourmet cooks overnight, but we need to start with the basics, always looking to our dinner guests for guidance.

Once you have the menu outlined, look around for the best sources for all your ingredients, the data. A supermarket, such as your hospital discharge dataset, is a good place to start; it is chock full of items that will give you data that will broadly cover providers who admit, attend, and consult on inpatients. However, you're going to need to be ready to visit niche specialty stores for those hard to shop for providers in Pathology, Radiology, Emergency Medicine, and Anesthesiology.

Over time, your menu will expand into the all-important privilege-based measures, and again you may need to venture out to special outlets for provider-based data, unique to certain specialties such as Gastroenterology, Cardiac Surgery, and Bariatrics.

Before you start cooking, check to be sure your ingredients are correct, fresh, free of impurities, and certainly not outdated. You will find that quality control in the kitchen is essential. You want your diners to enjoy their meals, and certainly not get sick!

So, get out the silverware and tablecloths, clean the kitchen, stock those shelves, heat up the oven, and let's serve some great profiles!

Why Professional Practice Profiles?

The modern history of measuring practitioner performance started a century ago, when Dr. Ernest A. Codman, a surgeon on the Harvard faculty, advocated for measuring and reporting surgical results, including long term follow-up. His efforts were roundly criticized by his peers, and so he left Massachusetts General Hospital to start his own small facility, dedicated to these "end results." However frustrating his early efforts were, they did lead to the creation of the American College of Surgeons in 1913, which, in turn, created a one page *Minimum Standard for Hospitals* in 1919. This document began to standardize the basic requirements associated with hospital and Medical Staff performance management ("American College of Surgeons," 2006). These standards prompted the creation of the Joint Commission on Accreditation of Hospitals in 1951; this entity is now known as The Joint Commission (TJC) ("History of The Joint Commission," 2015).

For much of the rest of the twentieth century, medicine was relatively simple and marginally effective; it was assumed that the best trained physicians provided the best care. As medicine became more specialized, the best care was assumed to be provided by specialists in referral centers doing the most advanced research. However, over the years, medicine has become both more effective and more complicated, with the results indicating that education and training are necessary, but not sufficient, to ensure safe and effective care by providers.

Healthcare continued to change in the second half of the twentieth century. During this time, accrediting organizations such as The Joint Commission required that Medical Staffs measure each provider's performance at the biennial reappointment cycle, with review and approval by the supervising physician, generally the department head, prior to reappointment. Although the review process itself ensured that at least a sample of credential files contained the proper profiles and signatures, there was no standard approach to these profiles. Further, the extent of review varied from hospital to hospital. In addition, there was no standard way to monitor provider performance in between the 2 year reappointments, aside from peer review of exceptional cases.

In 2007, The Joint Commission updated its Medical Staff standards to introduce the concept of professional practice evaluation that would be *ongoing* rather than *periodic*. This Ongoing Professional Practice Evaluation (OPPE) requires review of data on provider performance in between the standard 2 year reappointment cycles. The data must be reviewed more than once a year, usually every 6 or 8 months, to allow for performance improvement on a timely basis. Linked to OPPE is Focused Professional Practice Evaluation, or FPPE, which centers on measuring and improving performance in a focused manner, either at the time of initial appointment, replacing the older proctoring requirements, or when an OPPE triggers a more focused approach ("Standards FAQ details,"2013).

Considering that in 2015, 78% of U.S. hospitals were accredited by The Joint Commission ("Facts about hospital accreditation,"2015), it is no surprise that the OPPE requirement has driven the creation of practice profiles over the past 8 years. While The Joint Commission has been a leader in setting practice performance review standards, the concept has naturally spread outside the arena of hospital accreditation. A broad view of professional practice evaluation shows a number of growing uses:

- Evaluation of provider performance may function as part of ongoing monitoring associated with contracts or agreements between independent medical groups and hospitals. Although these contracts have been common for many years in the areas of Pathology, Radiology, and Emergency Medicine, similar contracts have been struck due to the evolution of Hospitalist provider practice; many of these include specific performance requirements.
- Evaluation of provider performance in outpatient settings, including measures of Volume and Performance for services including Outpatient Surgery, Cardiac Catheterization, and Endoscopic procedures, is fully expected and accepted in many situations. For staff model medical groups with dedicated inpatient facilities, inpatient and outpatient performance can be combined, serving multiple purposes.

Regardless of the reasons behind professional practice profiles and related performance evaluation/monitoring, the ultimate goal is to provide patient centered care that is: Safe, Effective, Efficient, Personalized, Timely, and Equitable ("Committee on quality health,"2001).

Who to Profile?

Broadly stated, at a minimum, profiles should be generated for licensed independent practitioners who are otherwise not evaluated through a human resources system. This includes physicians (MDs and DOs) and psychologists, as well as Advanced Practice Clinicians (APCs, including Certified Registered Nurse Anesthetists, Certified Nurse Midwives, Nurse Practitioners, and Physician Assistants) on the voluntary Medical Staffs of licensed hospitals in the United States. Note that this list may vary by state; likewise, variation may be specified in the hospital's Medical Staff bylaws, rules, and regulations.[1]

Until 2011, TJC-accredited hospitals could evaluate certain APCs through the Human Resources Department, depending on the practitioners' scope of practice. For many hospitals, this included employed Nurse Practitioners and Physician Assistants. However, in January 2011, TJC published a Joint Commission BoosterPak™, stating that those APCs who provide "medical level of care" as specified in the CMS CoPs must use the Medial Staff process for credentialing and privileging. The reader is encouraged to review both the relevant CMS CoPs and the standards for his/her accrediting organization for details ("The Joint Commission: Nurse practitioners," 2011).

What to Profile?

Provider profiles should reflect the performance of the provider in the areas in which he/she has privileges. A provider who has been credentialed and is a member of the Medical Staff but has no clinical privileges requires a minimal profile. Such a profile might include current licensure, continuing medical education, and attendance at meetings.

For all providers with privileges, profiles should reflect the fundamentals of their clinical activities in their areas of privileges, answering these basic questions:

---

[1]Many state Departments of Health have hospital licensing requirements far more specific than the common accrediting bodies, and, without a license, a hospital cannot keep its doors open. Be aware of your own state's requirements, and see how they address provider evaluation. Finally, always read your own Medical Staff bylaws, rules, and regulations to be sure they are up to date, and consistent with state and federal requirements, as well as those of your accrediting entity.

1. What does the provider have privileges to do?
2. Is he doing it?
3. Is he doing it well? (Smith & Pelletier, 2009)
4. Should he have done it?

The fourth question is difficult to answer, and not part of the traditional Medical Staff review. However, it is an important consideration as we move toward higher quality and greater efficiency. Multiple studies show that more care is not necessarily better care; further, unnecessary care not only raises the cost of care but increases the risk of adverse outcomes.

Less Can Be More

It seems intuitive that more of anything is better. Who would turn down more money, more food, more land, or a larger house? Knowing that a lack of medical care is not good, it seems that more medical care would be better. However, somewhere between scarcity and abundance, there is a sweet spot in the middle for medicine.

In June 2009, Atul Gawande, a Surgeon and public health researcher at Harvard, published a landmark article in *The New Yorker*, titled "The Cost Conundrum, What a Texas Town Can Teach Us about Health Care" (Gawande, 2009). He recounted a visit to McAllen, Texas, a border town not far from the Gulf Coast, where Medicare was spending almost twice the national average per patient, compared to a matched population in El Paso, due to overutilization of services. The article, with a rich mix of interviews and analysis, illustrated how more is not always better. Gawande went on to show how "more thinking and less testing" yields better outcomes, with the paradigm of the Mayo Clinic winning the day.

How can we apply this reality to provider profiling? One way is to consider appropriateness of care, and use best practice guidelines when building your measures, focusing on helping your colleagues do the right thing for the right patients at the right time (Fisher, 2003; Skinner, 2009).

To structure a privilege-based profile correctly, it is important to start with how the Medical Staff Office privileges and credentials a provider. Understanding this process will help you create a profile that flows out of the credentialing and privileging process. It will also help you locate the correct data sources for the Volume and Performance measures needed to track performance by privilege; see Chapter 6 for more information on data sources. Core privileging methods, when done effectively, create an excellent foundation for building performance profiles. For more detail on privileged-based measures, see Chapter 3.

The remainder of this volume fills in the details of *why, who,* and *what* to profile, beginning with Chapter 1, where we address current accreditation standards for acute care hospitals, including profile formats, number, and types of profiles expected. In Chapter 2, we focus on how to build Generic Profiles that cover all providers with privileges. In Chapter 3, we expand upon our profiles, adding indicators that reflect each provider's actual privileges. Chapter 4 covers the 4 unique specialties that challenge us because of their focused practices that are not well reflected in administrative datasets: Pathology, Radiology, Emergency Medicine, and Anesthesiology. Then, in Chapter 5, we cover profiles for Advanced Practice Clinicians.

Once we understand *what* we are building and for *whom*, we go on to explain *how*: in Chapter 6, we address data sources and checking data for Accuracy, Validity, and Reliability; in Chapter 7, we explain how to put together the team to accomplish initial profiling tasks and sustain profiles over time, so that our profiles become woven into the organization's structure. We wrap it all up with a summary in Chapter 8.

So let's head to the kitchen and get started!

Reference List:

"American College of Surgeons." (2006). Retrieved from https://www.facs.org/about%20acs/archives/pasthighlights/minimumhighlight January 12, 2015

"Committee on quality health care in America, Institute of Medicine." (2001). *Crossing the Quality Chasm: A New Health System for the 21st Century*, 41-56.

"Facts about hospital accreditation." (2015). The Joint Commission. Retrieved from http://www.jointcommission.org/facts_about_hospital_accreditation/

Fisher, E.S., Wennberg, D.E., Stukel, T.A., Gottlieb. D.J., Lucas, F.L., & Pinder, E.L. (2003). The implications of regional variations in Medicare spending, part 1: The content, quality, and accessibility of care. *Annals of Internal Medicine 138*: 273-287.

Gawande, A. (2009). The cost conundrum: What a Texas town can teach us about health care. *The New Yorker*, June 1, 2009. Retrieved from http://www.newyorker.com/magazine/2009/06/01/the-cost-conundrum

"History of The Joint Commission." (2015) The Joint Commission. Retrieved from http://www.jointcommission.org/about_us/history.aspx

Skinner, J. (2009). Is more care better care? *The New York Times*, Economix. Retrieved from http://economix.blogs.nytimes.com/2009/06/13/is-more-care-better-care/

Smith, M.A. & Pelletier, S. (2009). *Assessing the competency of low-volume practitioners*. HCPro: Marblehead, MA.

"Standards FAQ details." (2013). The Joint Commission. Retrieved from http://www.jointcommission.org/standards_information/jcfaqdetails aspx?StandardsFAQId=470&StandardsFAQChapterId=74

"The Joint Commission: Nurse Practitioners and Physician Assistants must be credentialed through the Medical Staff process." (2011). The National Law Review. Retrieved from http://www.natlawreview.com/article/joint-commission-nurse-practitioners-and-physician-assistants-must-be-credentialed-through-m

Chapter 1

Building Menus: Current Standards and Recommended Formats

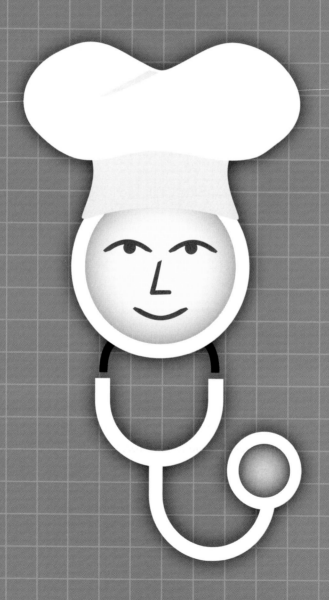

Starting with the Menu...

If you are going to cook a fine meal, you need to start with the menu, and understand who is coming to dinner.

The Joint Commission's tastes are relatively simple, but its surveyors are demanding, so be sure to include everything they expect. Your toughest guests are the Medical Staff members themselves – their tastes run to the gourmet and they are famous for sending plates back to the kitchen. Be sure they are involved in menu planning and be careful they don't ask for entrées you cannot provide. For more on the challenges of shopping for the data that will become your final meal, see Chapter 6.

All chefs know that presentation is important, so think ahead about how the meal will be arranged. This chapter will review 3 presentations or formats: The Joint Commission's Accreditation Council for Graduate Medical Education (ACGME) model; the the American Association for Physician Leadership/Greeley Model (see call-out box on American Association of Physician Leadership, this chapter); and an alternative offered as a best fit for commonly used measures and privilege-based profiles.

It is all right to start with a simple meal which appeals to everyone. However, in time, you will likely discover that special groups have special dietary needs, and the number of offerings available on the menu will need to grow to cover all of your specialties and their sets of privileges.

Bon appetité!

The first step in building provider profiles is to visualize the final product: what do you want the ideal profile to look like? Remember, your profiles need to meet the needs of the customers. Hence, we need to determine the answer to a vital question first: who are your customers?

In reality, your most important customers are Medical Staff members themselves: those being evaluated with the profiles; and the leaders of these departments or divisions who will use the profiles, both individually and in aggregate, to lead the improvement of the group. The profiles first and foremost must meet their needs, and provide useful information on the performance of the providers based on the privileges granted to them by the Medical Staff Office. The measures must be Relevant, Valid, Accurate, and Reliable. For more on ensuring the data is what you need, see Chapter 6.

Your secondary customers include any accrediting organizations or regulatory bodies that set standards for the inpatient Ongoing Professional Practice Evaluation (OPPE) process. With all due respect to the Medical Staff, let's begin with the standard-setting bodies, since they have created the most direction and content; starting here allows us to build a good foundation upon which the finer, more "gourmet" details can be added later.

A Short History of Deemed Status

When Medicare was passed into law in 1965, Congress had to determine which hospitals would be allowed to participate in the program. Rather than creating a new federal survey program, Congress passed this survey/ certification responsibility to the then dominant voluntary accreditation program, The Joint Commission on Accreditation of Hospitals (JCAHO). The law specified that any Joint Commission certified hospital had "deemed status" as a Medicare provider (Sprague, 2005). The Joint Commission continued to enjoy this designation unchallenged until 2008, when the Medicare Reform Bill specified that deeming authority required periodic application beginning in 2010. As of 2014, The Joint Commission, along with 3 other accrediting organizations (DNV-GL, HFAP, and CIHQ), continues to enjoy CMS deeming authority.

Hospitals are not required to be accredited by any of these organizations. They can request their needed certification directly from CMS, in which case they are surveyed on the CoPs by CMS representatives, generally members of the local state Department of Health.

It is fair to say that the dominant force in accreditation in the United States is the Centers for Medicare and Medicaid Services, or CMS, an operating division of the U.S. Department of Health and Human Services ("The Joint Commission," 2014). CMS has responsibility for administering the Medicare and Medicaid programs, including designating which facilities may participate in the programs, and assuring a minimal level of quality. It does this through a set of regulations called the Conditions of Participation (CoPs). To help facilitate this process, CMS has designated 4 accreditation programs for acute care hospitals as having standards and a survey process that meets or exceeds its CoPs. Hospitals that are accredited through these voluntary programs have "deemed status," which means they have met the CoPs and are therefore able to provide services, for which they are reimbursed, to Medicare/Medicaid recipients. Note that although regular CMS surveys are not required for accredited hospitals with deemed status, CMS does perform validation surveys for a sample of hospitals that have passed its surveys.

The CMS Conditions of Participation for hospitals includes a 21 page section on the Medical Staff, with a subsection that addresses appraisal by the Medical Staff of its members, Title 482.22(a)(1). See Appendix 1.1 for the full text. CMS expects an appraisal at least every 2 years, focused on each provider's scope of practice and privileges. Reviewing these standards may help you better understand the foundation for the standards of the 4 organizations with deeming authority.

As of this writing, the dominant voluntary accrediting organization in the U.S. is The Joint Commission, which has taken the lead in setting OPPE standards that not just meet but exceed the CMS Conditions of Participation.

For The Joint Commission, the practitioner profile is created as part of the broader Ongoing Professional Practice Evaluation (OPPE) process, as described in the Introduction. The provider profiles need to be reviewed every 6 to 8 months, and, of necessity, require data that reflects performance in the 6 to 8 months running up to the review. The measures should be trended over time to show changes in provider performance, and to provide comparisons to internal and external benchmarks to indicate the adequacy of this performance.

Any performance that falls below expectations must be addressed at the time of review, and depending on criteria set by the Medical Staff, may trigger a Focused Professional Practice Evaluation (FPPE). The Joint Commission is quite specific that the information resulting from the evaluation needs to be used to determine whether to continue, limit, or revoke any existing privileges at the time the information is reviewed. Record of any decisions needs to be included in each practitioner's credentials file upon review. Put another way, any major issues that might lead to a change in privileges, including suspension or revocation, need to be addressed when discovered as part of the OPPE cycle, not just at time of the biennial reappointment ("The Joint Commission," 2014).

The Joint Commission expects the OPPE process is clearly "defined," meaning a written policy should exist. This policy should detail who reviews the data, how often the data is reviewed, how the data is used to determine whether to continue, limit, or revoke a privilege, and how the data is incorporated into the credentials files. Note that there is no specific requirement that the data be continuously stored in the credentials files.

The types of data collected, as well as the measures that are built and tracked, must be defined by the Medical Staff Office, and approved by the Medical Staff as a whole. Data can come from a variety of sources, including individual chart review and direct observation or monitoring of diagnostic and treatment techniques, but must be customized to include Volume and performance in the areas of each provider's privileges. All practitioners must be reviewed, not just those with performance issues.

As noted above, 3 other organizations have CMS Deeming Authority. These include Det Norske Veritas-Germanischer Lloyd Healthcare (DNV-GL Healthcare), the American Osteopathic Association Healthcare Facilities Accreditation Program (AOA/HFAP), and the Center for Improvement in Healthcare Quality (CIHQ).

DNV-GL is an international classification society, with main locations in Norway and Germany. The company was formed in 2013 as a merger of Stiftelsen Det Norske Veritas (DNV) and Germanischer Lloyd (GL); it primarily operates as a ship and offshore classification society and a technical advisor to the global oil and gas industry ("DNV-GL Healthcare," 2014). In addition, it functions as a certification body, and, in this context, has created DNV-GL Healthcare, which runs a hospital accreditation program, the National Integrated Accreditation for Healthcare Organizations (NIAHO), which received CMS deeming authority in 2008. The NIAHO program integrates ISO-9001 with the Medicare Conditions of Participation. Hospitals have turned to DNV for their deeming needs primarily due to its integration with ISO-9001: 2008 standards, as well as it unique expertise associated with bio-risk, infection management, quality, and patient safety.

The current NIAHO guidelines, version 10.1, effective November 1, 2013, include a Medical Staff section with specific expectations on Performance Data, MS.9. These guidelines may be accessed online ("DNV: NIAHO Standards," 2013). Specifically:

Practitioner specific performance data is required to be evaluated, analyzed and appropriate action taken as necessary when variation is present and/or standard of care has not been met as determined by the medical staff. Performance data will be collected periodically within the reappointment period or as required as a part of the peer review process. This may include comparative and/or national data if available.

Areas required to be measured (as applicable) will include:
   SR.1 Blood use: (may include AABB transfusion criteria);
   SR.2 Prescribing of medications: Prescribing patterns, trends, errors and appropriateness of prescribing for Drug Use Evaluations;
   SR.3 Surgical Case Review: appropriateness and outcomes for selected high-risk procedures as defined by the medical staff;
   SR.4 Specific department indicators that have been defined by the medical staff;
   SR.5 Moderate Sedation Outcomes;
   SR.6 Anesthesia events;
   SR.7 Appropriateness of care for non-invasive procedures/interventions;
   SR.8 Utilization data;
   SR.9 Significant deviations from established standards of practice; and,
   SR.10 Timely and legible completion of patients' medical records.
   SR.11 Any variant should be analyzed for statistical significance.

These standards echo The Joint Commission's, especially in specifying that performance data 'will be collected periodically within the reappointment period.' With a reappointment period of 2 years, the frequency can be assumed to be every 6 to 8 months, same as TJC. Although no specific mention is made of measurement of performance by privileges, this can likely be assumed, especially with the wording of Surgical Care Review, with review of 'appropriateness and outcomes for selected high-risk procedures.' In addition, we may also note that there are criteria for assessing Appropriateness of Care.

The third organization with deeming authority is the Healthcare Facilities Accreditation Program (HFAP), created by the American Osteopathic Association in 1945 to review services provided by osteopathic hospitals. It gained deeming authority in 1966 by regulation rather than by statute[1], and provides accreditation services on a voluntary basis to all hospitals, allopathic or osteopathic. HFAP announced the addition of OPPE standards to its acute care manual in March 2014, effective January 1, 2015.

The HFAP standards align well with those established by The Joint Commission, specifically using the term Ongoing Professional Practice Evaluation. Further, they specifically call for a clearly defined plan for the evaluation of each practitioner's professional practice, approved by the Medical Staff, addressing details including identification of performance indicators specific to each department, data collection methods, individuals responsible for the data collection, methods of analysis, confidentiality and security of the data, and evaluation of low Volume practitioners. Of note is that these standards call for summarization of the data at least 3 times during each 2 year reappointment cycle. See Appendix 1.2 for details of the HFAP standards.

The fourth organization with deeming authority is the Center for Improvement in Healthcare Quality (CIHQ), having been certified by CMS in August 2013. Its manual of Accreditation Standards for Acute Care Hospitals, effective March 2014, includes a section within Medical Staff Bylaws that pertains to "periodic performance appraisal for members of the medical staff" that reflects the CMS Conditions of Participation:

MS-3: Medical Staff Bylaws (CIHQ, 2014, p. 7):

The medical staff shall establish, adopt and enforce bylaws, rules, regulations, and policies to carry out its responsibilities. The bylaws (including any revisions) must be approved by the governing body. At a minimum, the bylaws must address: …

---

[1]Deeming status for The Joint Commission, then known as the Joint Commission for Accreditation of Hospitals (JCAH), was granted in 1965 by statute, meaning that it was written into the original Medicare law. HFAP was granted deeming authority in 1966 by regulation, meaning that it was written into the regulations written to implement the law (Sprague, 2005).

E. The criteria and process for periodic performance appraisals for members of the medical staff, including those who have not provided patient care within the organization or who has not provided care for which he/she is privileged to provide during the appropriate evaluation time frames.

- *In developing criteria, the medical staff should consider the following: current work practice, special training, quality of specific work, patient outcomes, education, maintenance of continuing education, adherence to medical staff rules, certifications, appropriate licensure, and currency of compliance with licensure requirements*

As with the CMS CoPs, the frequency of review is at least biennial. There is no mention of "ongoing" review, or specific frequency as seen in the TJC, DNV, and HFAP standards.

To consider this information collectively, start by realizing the following. CMS calls for "periodic" review of providers, and states this has to occur at least every 2 years unless mandated more frequently by the state. The Joint Commission calls for "OPPE" on an ongoing basis, defined as more frequently than yearly. DNV calls for data to be collected "periodically within the reappointment period [which is 2 years] or as required by the peer review process." HFAP borrows the TJC language of OPPE (standard effective January 2015) and states that the process is "ongoing" and "data will be collected… and summarized at least three times during each two year appointment cycle" ("Healthcare Facilities Accreditation Program," 2014, p. 3-50). Further, CIHQ mirrors the CMS CoPs, but does not require provider reports more often than every 2 years.

Regardless of which accrediting organization your hospital uses, here are a few guiding principles:

- The provider profiling standards for all organizations with deeming authority are based on the CMS Conditions of Participation. Be familiar with the CMS standards, as well those that may be unique to your accreditation organization.
- Read carefully the specific standards for your accrediting organization, as they vary by organization, and may be more specific and detailed than the CMS standards.

- Check your state Department of Health to see if there are local standards you need to add to your list.
- Provider profiling/OPPE is by and for the Medical Staff; every hospital needs a written Medical Staff policy that covers the basics, with additional detail to satisfy the accrediting body, and, as applicable, the state or states in which the hospital operates. Some of the accrediting organizations' requirements exceed the basic CMS standards.
- Keep focused on privileges – "what can the provider do, did she do it, and did she do it well?" (Smith, 2009). Consider adding appropriateness criteria, addressing the question: "Should she have done it?"
- If your hospital has elected to forego voluntary accreditation and go directly to CMS and state surveys, look directly to the CMS Conditions of Participation.

As noted earlier, your most important customers are the Medical Staff members themselves: those being evaluated by the profiles and the leaders of the departments or divisions who will use the profiles both individually and in aggregate to lead the improvement of the groups. Make sure that these vital individuals are involved in developing both the basic policy on provider profiling, and the profiles themselves. Remember that the policies, plans, and processes need to come from the Medical Staff; all measures must likewise be approved by the Medical Staff.

It is helpful to provide Medical Staff leadership with draft profiles, and ask them to "mark them up," removing irrelevant measures, adding metrics specific to their specialties focused on granted privileges, working within the context of the foundational requirements of your accrediting organization. It is easier to review a draft in hand than to come up with a profile de novo. We will go into more detail on this process in Chapter 7.

Start with a Draft

draft: noun. A version of something (such as a document) that you make before you make the final version; a preliminary version ("Draft," 2015).

When seeking a useful, effective provider profile, it is helpful to create a draft profile even though you know it is not your final product. The draft establishes a place to start, and functions as the centerpiece for conversations among members of the Medical Staff, the Medical Staff Office, and other departments. Drafts are especially helpful when working with providers. It gives them a document to which they may react; even if that reaction is not the most positive (this can happen!), It often results in new content, as in "no, no — do it this way!"

It may be helpful to buy a big rubber stamp that says "DRAFT," and stamp your working documents liberally with it, to emphasize that each is not final, but rather a working document that is intended to change over time.

In this spirit, the profiles that are offered in this volume are also drafts; they are suggested starting points. Although we are offering the best place to start based on our collective knowledge and experience, we are positive that our readers can take this starting point and make it better.

Remember:
No drafts are perfect, but all drafts are helpful!

Formatting Provider Profiles: Available Choices

The way the profiles are organized makes a difference. Grouping measures that are related or similar often makes the entire profile easier to read and understand; certain measures make more sense when grouped together. Also, grouping allows the reviewer, be it the provider himself, or his chief, to extract more information about performance by examining related measures together.

When The Joint Commission first rolled out its OPPE standards in 2008, it recommended that the measures for provider profiles be grouped into 6 categories, based on the 6 domains of clinical competency created by the

Accreditation Council for Graduate Medical Education (ACGME), as part of a multiyear process of restructuring its accreditation system to be based on educational outcomes (Nasca, Philibert, Brigham, & Flynn, 2012). The 6 ACGME domains for residents in training are:

Patient Care: Residents must be able to provide patient care that is compassionate, appropriate, and effective for the treatment of health problems and the promotion of health.

Medical Knowledge: Residents must be able to demonstrate knowledge about established and evolving biomedical, clinical, and cognate (e.g., epidemiological and social-behavioral) sciences and the application of this knowledge to patient care.

Practice-Based Learning and Improvement: Residents must be able to investigate and evaluate their patient care practices, appraise and assimilate scientific evidence, and improve their patient care practices.

Interpersonal and Communication Skills: Residents must be able to demonstrate interpersonal and communication skills that result in effective information exchange and teaming with patients, patients' families, and professional associates.

Professionalism: Residents must be able to demonstrate a commitment to carrying out professional responsibilities, adherence to ethical principles, and sensitivity to a diverse patient population.

Systems-Based Practice: Residents must be able to demonstrate an awareness of and responsiveness to the larger context and system of health care and the ability to effectively call on system resources to provide care that is of optimal value.

As of this printing, it is common for TJC accredited hospitals to use these 6 domains to arrange performance measures. As noted earlier, it often helps to group related measures together, so this approach is helpful, and meets TJC's recommendation.

However, some objections to this method have been raised. A primary objection to this format as applied to provider profiles is that it was designed for residents in training who are constantly being supervised or otherwise monitored, not for providers practicing independently. The categories lend themselves to metrics that assume either direct observation or the ability to otherwise demonstrate or show a skill or ability.

Nevertheless, the measures that are amenable to provider profiling can be grouped into these 6 categories, plus additional categories for Volume and Acuity. The following is offered as an example of provider metrics grouped into the ACGME domains:

Volume:
- Counts of Patient Encounters as Attending, Surgeon (Proceduralist), and Consultant

Acuity:
- Average Case Mix Index (CMI)

Patient Care:
- Mortality Counts and Rates; Complication Rates; Outcomes Based on Privileges

Medical Knowledge:
- Core Measure Compliance; CME Activity

Interpersonal and Communication:
- Patient Satisfaction Results
- Internal Satisfaction Surveys

Systems-Based Practice:
- Average Length of Stay (ALOS)
- Readmission Rates
- Adjusted Cost per Case

Professionalism:
- Patient Complaints (Peer Reviewed)
- Timeliness and Completion of Operative Notes, Discharge Summaries
- Validated Non-Compliance with Medical Staff Rules and Regulations

Practice-Based Learning and Improvement:
- Peer Reviewed Cases

A full model of suggested indicators grouped by the 6 competencies is shown in Table 1.1.

A second format has been developed by the American College of Physician Executives, now known as the American Association for Physician Leadership, for use in its actions associated with managing physician performance in group practices. This format has been adopted by The Greeley Company for use by Medical Staffs (Marder et. al, 2007). It defines 6 performance dimensions as follows:

- Technical Quality
- Service Quality
- Relationships
- Citizenship
- Patient Safety/Patient Rights
- Resource Use

Tip: *If you are TJC accredited but decide to use a non-ACGME format, create a sample crosswalk for use at the time of your survey to demonstrate to TJC that you understand the ACGME format. This crosswalk will also illustrate that the measures on your profiles cover the 6 domains.*

American Association for Physician Leadership

In 2014, American College of Physician Executives (ACPE) became the American Association for Physician Leadership. Founded in 1975, this organization saw the need to change its name as a response to the great developments in healthcare that currently highlight the need for physician leadership. Per the new organization's website, "The organization's new identity better reflects the significant role the association will continue to play in helping physicians from all backgrounds and in all types of positions realize their leadership potential" ("American College of Physician Executives," 2014).

As an alternative to the ACGME and AAPL formats, we offer a third format, with mapping to the ACGME competencies, as an approach that may, in fact, be a better fit for the cascading set of profiles outlined in this chapter.

Further, we believe this format will better serve the user as we move toward privilege-based profiles. In the next chapter, we will build a sample Generic Profile using this format. It is offered as a draft with which to start, and then revise/fine-tune as appropriate.

We believe that this alternative deserves a name, something more than "a third format." Therefore, we have named our format Talis Qualis, abbreviated simply as TQ, as a nod to the same Latin phrase, meaning 'just as such.'

To us, Talis Qualis is 'just as such,' in that it is a start—something meant to be modified per your discretion and needs. TQ is not intended to be a stagnant, impenetrable profile format without flexibility; to the contrary, it is a proposal intended to grow and develop with your organizational needs and demands. At the same time, however, it is set up with reason behind its design; you will note that metrics are grouped logically and with forethought. Likewise, it is the result of experience—perhaps not at your hospital, with your Medical Staff, but with many hospitals and Medical Staffs across the country. Further, TQ is the result of assessing what is working, what isn't working, and what is missing from formats that have been used and modified time and again.

The TQ format (Table 1.2) includes the following major headings or domains:

- Volume
- Acuity
- Clinical Outcomes
- Efficiency
- Processes of Care
- Privilege-Based Measures
    o Privilege 1
    o Privilege 2
    o Privilege ...
- Patient Satisfaction
- Citizenship
- Reviews

We begin with the basics, Volume based on Discharges, Procedures, and/or Visits; we then move to measures of Acuity for the population served.

Note that TQ reflects our belief that Volume is the first and probably most important metric. If a provider has low Volume, the patient population of interest will not be, in many cases, large enough for the remainder of the metrics to be meaningful (Dimick et. al, 2004; Fetterolf et. al, 2008). Low Volume practitioners need to be profiled on a limited set of metrics, and should logically have a limited set of privileges. A profile designed for the highest Volume, highest Acuity providers will be meaningless for the low Volume doctor. In addition, research shows Volume correlates with positive outcomes, so understanding up front the provider's Volume is important (Livingston et. al, 2010).

Acuity, quantified via Case-Mix Index (CMI), is measured as the average of the MS-DRG, or APR-DRG, Relative Weights for the population of interest. If the Volume is high, but Acuity low, the practitioner may be providing a high level of care that is not needed for this "less sick" population. Alternatively, he may be having difficulty with appropriate chart documentation, leading to an average Relative Weight that is lower than expected for the population.

Once we have Volume and Acuity measures in hand, the next set of metrics relates to the Clinical Outcomes of the encounter, including Risk-Adjusted Mortality and Complications. Again, these measures have more meaning as a provider's Volume increases. For more on Risk Adjustment, see Chapter 6.

The next set of measures relates to Efficiency of Care, which highlights how resources are being used to care for the population. Metrics here may include Length of Stay, Acuity-Adjusted Cost per Case, and Readmissions. Note that we have included Readmissions here because they may be looked at as a form a re-work, as well as a potential quality issue. You may choose to likewise include them here, in Efficiency of Care; logical arguments may be made, however, for them to be included in Volume, Processes of Care, or other categories.

Moving along, we next include Processes of Care measures, considering what providers do to improve final Outcomes. Core Measures and other best practice measures can be located here, along with measures of Drug and Blood Utilization.

All of the above metrics pertain to all providers with privileges covered by a profile, and would include the provider's Total Patient Population, regardless of diagnosis or procedure performed.

The next section organizes all of the measures grouped by the provider's privileges. For example, for a Gastroenterologist, Upper Endoscopy may be a privilege that would have its own heading; this heading would include Volume, Acuity, Processes of Care, Outcomes, and Efficiency – all for that specific procedure. This structure allows the provider and his chief to quickly review his performance for this privilege, without having to search the entire profile, or request a special report. In addition, note that we believe that this section should include the provider's main procedures, especially those that are high Volume, high risk, and/or problem-prone. For more on building privilege-based measures, see Chapter 3.

Once we have delineated the provider's main privileges, the next section is Patient Satisfaction, the patients' perceptions of their care. These measures may come from the hospital's patient satisfaction surveys, provided that the information has accurate attribution of the attributed provider, be he/she the Attending, Principal Procedure Provider, or other identified provider.

Next is the broad category of Citizenship; it encompasses all the things that providers should do as part of a community of providers. Measures here may include: Timely Completion of Medical Records; Compliance with Medical Staff Bylaws, Rules, and Regulations; Results of Internal Staff Surveys; Participation in Medical Staff Committees; and Participation in Training of Residents. We have also included CME Credits here, on the assumption that staying current with education and maintaining certification is part of the provider's obligation to his practice community, as well as to his patients.

The final section is the broad category of Reviews. Here are the metrics related to Review of Cases by Peers (Peer Review), with the outcomes of these reviews. If you want to track Risk Management Issues, they can go here; indicators could include Claims Pending, Claims Settled, and so forth. A review of any specific issues related to Invasive Procedures, Conscious Sedation, Infection Control, Blood Usage, and/or Pharmacy and Therapeutics also falls into this category. In addition, we suggest including a Count of the Number of Reviews Performed with Outcome of the Review, per the Medical Staff policy.

In Table 1.2, suggested mapping of these categories to the ACGME 6 competencies is provided.

One of the advantages of our TQ format is that it creates logical domains that are not only helpful one by one for review, but also allows for comparison of the domains to each another, which, in turn, creates additional information. For example:

- Processes of Care may be compared to Clinical Outcomes. If all Processes of Care requirements are being met, one would expect the risk-adjusted Outcomes to be average or better. If they are not, then the Process measures may not be Valid, or the Outcome Adjustment may not be Accurate.

- Efficiency can be compared to Outcomes, and to Volume. Research has shown that high Volume hospitals and high Volume providers tend to have better Outcomes (Birkmeyer, 2002 & 2003; Livingston, 2010). If a high Volume provider has problems with Efficiency measures, specific drill down to cases and processes may help to improve his Efficiency.

- Privilege-Based measures address the key question of if a provider should continue to have a specific privilege, and if a Focused Professional Practice Evaluation (FPPE) is warranted. Grouping all metrics by privilege provides the best view of performance by privilege category, and may find Outcome or Efficiency issues that would otherwise be buried in the global measures for high Volume providers.

- Patient Satisfaction scores should correlate with the other measures. If not, the provider may have high technical skill, but need improvement in his relationships with his patients.

- The Number and Results of Reviews should correlate with all the other measures. If a provider has issues with Outcomes, Efficiency, Processes of Care, Patient Satisfaction, and/or Citizenship, one would expect an appropriate Number of Reviews, with action plans. If the numbers of Reviews are low, or non-existent, then the Review process comes into question. In turn, if all the metrics look good, but there are many Reviews, one should consider why this provider is being reviewed to this degree and quantity.

This ability to link the domains is similar to the process described by Kaplan and Norton in their book *The Balanced Scorecard, Translating Strategy into Action* (1996).

Building Profiles: How Many Do You Need?

Once we understand why we are building profiles, our audience, and the format we are using, the next question is how many profiles should we build? Before we answer, or attempt to answer this question, we have work to do in regard to some basic assumptions. First, let's assume that all members of a clinical division or department with similar privileges share the same profile. This creates standardization within a division or department, which is important to create a "level playing field" at the time of OPPE review. It also facilitates the aggregation of the data for evaluation by division, which is important for specialties such as Hospitalist Medicine, where attending attribution is a challenge.

Now, let's also realize that for a 200-400 bed hospital, with multiple specialties and Advanced Practice Clinicians (APCs, including PAs, NPs, CRNAs, and CNMs; see Chapter 5 for more information), the total number of unique department/specialty profiles may expand up to 50. See Table 1.3 for a list of possible profiles for a large multi-specialty hospital.

Although you may need to reach this number as a final goal, we all understand that we have to start somewhere. In our experience, it is best to start with a Generic Profile that covers the basics for all providers with privileges; after we have established a base Generic Profile, we can branch off, adding distinct profiles for specialties depending on their privilege sets. Put another way, we start with a base meal, and add side dishes depending on the special needs of diners.

At the outset, a set of profiles might look like this:

- A base Generic Profile that covers the basics for all providers with privileges who see inpatients as an Attending or Consultant
- Profiles for 4 specialties with practices that are sufficiently unique to require special attention for both measure construction and data sources:
  - o Pathology
  - o Radiology
  - o Emergency Medicine
  - o Anesthesiology

Once we have addressed our foundation, the next step is to add measures to the Generic Profile to create 2 broad but distinct categories, as follows:

- A Surgical Profile that adds measures for Volume and Performance by Procedure Provider, to begin to reflect performance of providers with interventional privileges. This profile will broadly cover Surgeons regardless of their specialty, and providers in interventional specialties, such as Invasive Cardiology.
- An Internal Medicine/Hospitalist Medicine/Pediatric profile that adds measures with greater diagnostic specificity, reflecting patient mix, CMS/TJC Core Measures appropriate to these specialties, and drug prescribing patterns.

At this point, we have 7 profiles that cover all physician providers with privileges:

1. Base Generic
2. Generic Medical
3. Generic Surgical
4. Pathology
5. Radiology
6. Emergency Medicine
7. Anesthesiology

With use of the Generic Medical and Generic Surgical Profiles, the base Generic Profile may become redundant and may be retired.

The next step is to look at the Advanced Practice Clinicians, and begin to create profiles to address their performance. This is a challenge, but you can be successful; see Chapter 5.

Once you have the 7 profiles as listed above working well, begin to create more specific profiles based on clusters of shared privileges. Examples include:

- Orthopedics
- Pediatrics
- Neonatology

- General Surgery
- Surgical Specialties (Urology, Head and Neck, Vascular, Cardiac)
- Hospitalists, including Internal Medicine
- Cardiology
- Critical Care/Pulmonary
- Gastroenterology
- Behavioral Health/Psychiatry
- Rehabilitation/Physical Medicine

Look carefully at your departments and divisions to see if the current organizational structure aligns with privilege sets. In some cases, agreement will be evident; for example, in Gastroenterology, the majority of department members will share the same privileges, with a few members also doing advanced specialized procedures, such as Endoscopic Ultrasound, Manometry, and/or Capsule Endoscopy. In this case, a single profile with provision for special procedures will suffice. In other departments, there may be more variation in privileging. For example, in the Department of General Surgery, you may have groups of practitioners who cluster around shared privileges, such as Bariatric Surgery or Breast Surgery. The profiles associated with a General Surgery Department need to center on the privilege clusters, even if these do not correspond to the formal administrative department or departments. We realize that at times, a lack of alignment may be seen as problematic, but our experience tells us that a privilege-based structure is most often superior than one based on departmental headings alone. See Table 1.3 for examples of privilege-based profiles that may all fall into the Department of Surgery.

Once again, we want to stress the fact that with any of these profiles, but especially those that are specialty oriented, there is value in viewing them both by individual provider, and aggregated by the specialty. An aggregate profile is especially helpful when the division's providers work as a team, such as Hospitalists or Intensivists, and the status as "Attending" is therefore shared. Some of the best performance improvement work can be done as the team looks at its performance collectively, while the individual provider profiles meet review and reappointment requirements and aid in individual performance improvement initiatives.

██ Summary

At the outset of this chapter, we came to an understanding of who is coming to dinner; that is, we agreed about who will be using the profiles being built, including accrediting bodies and the Medical Staff. Next, we looked at the menu itself, visualizing what the profiles will look like, and how they will be formatted. Finally, we reviewed how many profiles we will need, remembering to start slowly, and build as we gain more experience, adding metrics for providers by their privileges. In the next chapter, we will build our first profile, a generic foundation for any member of the Medical Staff with privileges.

Reference List:

"About DNV-GL." (2014). DNV-GL. Retrieved from http://dnvgl.com/about-dnvgl/default.aspx

"Accreditation requirements – Acute care manual updates." (2014). Healthcare Facilities Accreditation Program. Retrieved from http://hfap.org/blog/?p=9961

"The American College of Physician Executives is becoming the American Association for Physician Leadership." (2014). American Association for Physician Leadership. Retrieved from http://www.physicianleaders.org/join/about-us/our-new-name

"DNV-NIAHO standards." (2013) DNV-GL. Retrieved from http://public.verge-`so lutions.com/VSuiteHelp/default htm?turl=Documents%2Fdnvniahostandards.htm

"Healthcare Facilities Accreditation Program (HFAP) Accreditation Requirements for Acute Care Hospitals." (2014). Retrieved from http://aoa-opan.informz. net/aoa-opan/data/images/Acute%20manual%20update%20March%20 2014/031501.pdf

Birkmeyer, J.D., Siewers, A.E., Finlayson, E.V., Stukel, T.A., Lucas, F.L., Batista, I., ...Wennberg, D.E. (2002). Hospital volume and surgical mortality in the United States. *New England Journal of Medicine*, 346: 1128-1137.

Birkmeyer, J.D., Stukel, T.A., Siewers, A.E., Goodney, P.P., Wennberg, D.E., & Lucas, F.L. (2003). Surgeon volume and operative mortality in the United States. *New England Journal of Medicine*, 349(22): 2117-2127

"Center for Improvement in Healthcare Quality." (2014). Accreditation standards for acute care hospitals, effective October 2014. Retrieved from http://www.cihq.org/home.asp

Dimick, J.B., Welch, H.G., & Birkmeyer, J.D. (2004). Surgical mortality as an indicator of hospital quality. *The Journal of the American Medical Association*, 292: 847-851.

"DNV-GL Healthcare." (2014) DNV-GL Healthcare. Retrieved from http://dnvglhealthcare.com/

"Draft." (2015). Merriam-Webster. Retrieved from http://www.merriam-webster.com/dictionary/draft

Fetterolf, D. & Tucker, T.L. (2008). Assessment of medical management outcomes in small populations. *Population Health Management*, 11: 233-239.

Kaplan, R.S., & Norton, D.P. (1996). Linking balanced scorecard measures to your strategy. *The Balanced Scorecard, Translating Strategy into Action*. Boston, MA: Harvard Business School Press.

Livingston, E.H., & Cao, J. (2010). Procedure volume as a predictor of surgical outcomes. *The Journal of the American Medical Association*, (304): 95-97.

Marder, R., Smith, M., Smith, M., & Searcy, V. (2007). *Measuring physician competency, how to collect, assess, and provide performance data.* (2nd edition). Marblehead, MA: HCPro, Inc.

Nasca, T.J., Philibert, I., Brigham, T., & Flynn, T.C. (2012). The next GME accreditation system-rationale and benefits. *New England Journal of Medicine*, (366): 1051-1056.

"National Integrated Accreditation for Healthcare Organizations (NIAHO) interpretive guidelines and surveyor guidance, Version 10.1, effective November 1, 2012." (2012). DNV Healthcare Inc., Milford, OH. Retrieved from http://dnvgl-healthcare.com/registration

"Operating divisions." (2014). U.S. Department of Health and Human Services. Retrieved from http://www.hhs.gov/about/foa/opdivs/index.html

"Reform of hospital and critical access hospital Conditions of Participation." (2014). Centers for Medicare and Medicaid Services. Retrieved from http://www.cms.gov/Regulations-and-Guidance/Legislation/CFCsAndCoPs/Hospitals.html

Smith M.A., & Pellitier S. (2009). *Assessing the Competency of Low-Volume Practitioners* (2nd Edition). Marblehead, MA: HCPro.

Sprague, L. (2005). Hospital oversight in Medicare: Accreditation and deeming authority. National Health Policy Forum Issue Brief No. 802, The George Washington University, Washington, DC. Retrieved from http://www.nhpf.org/library/issue-briefs/IB802_Accreditation_05-06-05.pdf

"The Joint Commission FAQ page." (2014). The Joint Commission. Retrieved from http://www.jointcommission.org/about/JointCommissionFaqs.aspx

Appendix 1.1

The most recent CMS conditions of participation (CoPs) for hospitals may be found on the CMS website.

http://www.cms.gov/Regulations-and-Guidance/Guidance/Manuals/index.html

The CMS standards, current as of March 21, 2014, that pertain to provider profiling are included here for reference:

§482.22(a)(1) - The medical staff must periodically conduct appraisals of its members. Interpretive Guidelines §482.22(a)(1)

The medical staff must at regular intervals appraise the qualifications of all practitioners appointed to the medical staff/granted medical staff privileges. In the absence of a State law that establishes a timeframe for periodic reappraisal, a hospital's medical staff must conduct a periodic appraisal of each practitioner. CMS recommends that an appraisal be conducted at least every 24 months for each practitioner.

The purpose of the appraisal is for the medical staff to determine the suitability of continuing the medical staff membership or privileges of each individual practitioner, to determine if that individual practitioner's membership or privileges should be continued, discontinued, revised, or otherwise changed.

The medical staff appraisal procedures must evaluate each individual practitioner's qualifications and demonstrated competencies to perform each task or activity within the applicable scope of practice or privileges for that type of practitioner for which he/she has been granted privileges. Components of practitioner qualifications and demonstrated competencies would include at least: current work practice, special training, quality of specific work, patient outcomes, education, maintenance of continuing education, adherence to medical staff rules, certifications, appropriate licensure, and currency of compliance with licensure requirements.

In addition to the periodic appraisal of members, any procedure/task/activity/ privilege requested by a practitioner that goes beyond the specified list of privileges for that particular category of practitioner requires an appraisal by the medical staff and approval by the governing body. The appraisal must consider evidence of qualifications and competencies specific to the nature of the request. It must also consider whether the activity/task/procedure is one that the hospital can support when it is conducted within the hospital. Privileges cannot be granted for tasks/procedures/activities that are not conducted within the hospital, regardless of the individual practitioner's ability to perform them.

After the medical staff conducts its reappraisal of individual members, the medical staff makes recommendations to the governing body to continue, revise, discontinue, limit, or revoke some or all of the practitioner's privileges, and the governing body takes final appropriate action.

A separate credentials file must be maintained for each medical staff member. The hospital must ensure that the practitioner and appropriate hospital patient care areas/departments are informed of the privileges granted to the practitioner, as well as of any revisions or revocations of the practitioner's privileges. Furthermore, whenever a practitioner's privileges are limited, revoked, or in any way constrained, the hospital must, in accordance with State and/or Federal laws or regulations, report those constraints to the appropriate State and Federal authorities, registries, and/or data bases, such as the National Practitioner Data Bank.

Survey Procedures §482.22(a)(1)
- Determine whether the medical staff has a system in place that is used to reappraise each of its current members and their qualifications at regular intervals, or, if applicable, as prescribed by State law.
- Determine whether the medical staff by-laws identify the process and criteria to be used for the periodic appraisal.
- Determine whether the criteria used for reevaluation comply with the requirements of this section, State law and hospital bylaws, rules, and regulations.
- Determine whether the medical staff has a system to ensure that practitioners seek approval to expand their privileges for tasks/activities/procedures that go beyond the specified list of privileges for their category of practitioner.
- Determine how the medical staff conducts the periodic appraisals of any current member of the medical staff who has not provided patient care at the hospital or who has not provided care for which he/she is privileged to patients at the hospital during the appropriate evaluation time frames. Is this method in accordance with State law and the hospital's written criteria for medical staff membership and for granting privileges?

Appendix 1.2

Healthcare Facilities Accreditation Program Updates:
http://www.hfap.org/blog/?p=9961, posted March 11, 2014:

03.15.01 Ongoing Professional Practice Evaluation.
Ongoing professional practice evaluation (OPPE) information is factored into
the decision to maintain existing privilege(s), to revise existing privilege(s), and/
or to revoke an existing privilege prior to or at the time of renewal. Effective:
January 1, 2015

The Medical Staff have a process to monitor the competency of its members.
Through an ongoing review of performance measurements, negative trends
are tracked and trended in a manner that allows the leadership to identify
performance issues and implement strategies that will effect change. Prospective
and real-time evaluation is important to ensure the delivery of safe and
competent care.

The Medical Staff develop an ongoing professional practice evaluation plan that
is applicable to all practitioners with privileges granted by the governing body.

The plan for the evaluation of each practitioner's professional practice is clearly
defined. This medical staff approved plan addresses each of the following:
1. Reasons for ongoing professional practice performance evaluations
2. Identification of performance indicators specific to each department of the
   medical staff
3. Data collection methods
4. Individual(s) responsible for data collection
5. Sources of data, e.g., medical records
6. Frequency of data collection
7. Methods for evaluation and analysis of data
8. Confidentiality and security of data
9. Individuals that may access individual practitioner's professional practice data
10. Explanation that data will be used as a measure of competency and will be
    reviewed at time of reappointment to determine eligibility
11. Evaluation of low volume practitioners
12. Triggers for additional, focused monitoring

Processes are established to ensure the confidentiality and security of the Ongoing
professional practice evaluation data. The medical staff identify individuals that
may access and review the data, for example:

- Respective department chair
- Credentials committee
- Medical Executive Committee (MEC)
- Special committees
- Chief of Staff
- Chief Medical Officer / Vice President of Medical Affairs (VPMA)
- Personnel working in the Medical Staff Office, Quality Department, or Medical Records Department

Data will be collected on an ongoing basis and summarized at least three (3) times during each two-year appointment cycle. It is recommended that individual data reports be distributed to the practitioners.

When possible, data collection systems that are currently in place should be accessed to measure individual practitioner outcomes. Electronic billing data, for example, often provides information according to the admitting and attending physician, primary surgeon, consultants and other practitioners. Billing data, however, may have limited usefulness for the mid-level providers, as traditional coding practices may not identify this group of practitioners.

At least every two (2) years, the Medical Staff identify and approve performance measurements that are specific to the services provided by the practitioners. Examples of performance measures include:

1. Administrative Data
   - # Admissions
   - # Consultations
   - # Weeks on Surgery Suspension List
   - Medical record delinquency rate
2. Clinical Indicators
   - Core measures (Heart Failure, Acute Myocardial Infarction, Pneumonia, Stroke, and etc.)
   - SCIP (Surgical Care Improvement Project)
   - Returns to surgery
   - Surgical infection rate
   - Procedural complication data
   - Administration of corticosteroids within 24 hours of admission for asthma
   - Cesarean section births, not medically necessary
   - Turnaround time for simple / complicated autopsy reports

The Medical Staff determine data to be collected for the mid-level practitioners (NP, PA, CRNA, CNM) that are relevant to their practice.

Table 1.1 A provider profile in the format of the ACGME 6 competencies:

CATEGORY	MEASURE
Volume	
	Volume as Attending: All Patients
	Volume as Attending (Acute Care)
	Volume as Attending Outpatient/Short Stay
	Volume as Consultant: Total Inpatients Seen in Consultation
	Volume as Consultant: Acute Care Only
	Volume of Outpatient Procedures/Short Stay
	Volume: Total Procedures Performed, Acute, Non-Acute, Short Stay, Outpatient
	Volume as Principal Procedure Provider (Acute Care)
	Volume of Procedures as Procedure Provider
Acuity	
	Case Mix Index (CMI) as Attending (Acute Care)
	Average CMI as Principal Procedure Provider (Acute Care)
Systems-Based Practice	
	Average Length of Stay (LOS) as Attending (Acute Care)
	Average Length of Stay (LOS) as Principal Procedure Provider (Acute Care)
	% Readmission within 30 Days as Attending (Acute Care)
	% Return to Surgery as Principal Procedure Provider (Acute Care)
	Cost/RW as Attending
	Cost/RW as Principal Procedure Provider
Patient Care	
	Deaths as Attending (Acute Care)
	Deaths as Principal Procedure Provider (Acute Care)
	Mortality Rate as Attending (Unadjusted, Acute Care)
	Mortality Rate as Principal Procedure Provider (Unadjusted-Acute Care)
	Mortality Rate of Pts w/ Major Complications as Attending
	Total Pending Claims
	Claims Settled
	Pending Judgments
	Rare Events as Attending (Acute Care)
	Rare Event, Death Following a Procedure as PPP (Acute Care)

DATA-DRIVEN HEALTHCARE IMPROVEME

Condition Good

Location Aisle 7 Bay 7 Shelf 2 item 463

Description Used book in good condition. May have some wear to binding, spine, cover, and pages. Some light markings/writing may be present. May have some stickers and/or sticker residue present. If applicable, book's access code, disc, and/or accessories are not included unless otherwise specified. All items shipped Monday - Friday. Fast shipping - Books ship in envelope.

Source 080 - eBooks
SKU 352BVG0O0NZA
ISIN 0984205136
ISBN 0984205136

CATEGORY	MEASURE
Medical Knowledge	
	Appropriate Use of Blood and Blood Products
	Core Measures - AMI, CHF, SCIP, PN
Interpersonal and Communication Skills	
	Reported Events
Practice-Based Learning and Improvement; Professionalism	
Peer Review/Case Review	
	Total Cases Peer Reviewed
	Total Cases: Care Excellent
	Total Cases: Appropriate Care
	Total Cases: Opportunity for Improvement
	Total Cases: System Opportunity for Improvement
Quality Improvement	
	Invasive Procedure Issues
	Infection Control Issues
	Blood Usage Issues
	P and T Issues
	Conscious Sedation Issues
	Restraint Issues

Table 1.2 Proposed TQ Format Profile:

TQ CATEGORY	MEASURE SUMMARY	RATIONALE	ACGME CATEGORY
Volume	Volume of Discharges as Attending, Procedures Provider, Consultant	How many patients is the provider seeing over time, and in what role? Volume correlates with Positive Outcomes.	Patient Care
Acuity	Average CMI by MS-DRG and APR-DRG, as Attending, Procedure Provider	How "sick" are these patients? Their levels of Acuity correlate with resource use, and is helpful in identifying where the provider is in relationship to the Volume. High Volume and high Acuity might be a tip off to unnecessary use of resources, which creates its own quality issues.	Patient Care
Clinical Outcome	Clinical Outcomes of Care Including Mortality, Complications, and Other Events, Risk-Adjusted When Possible	Once we know Volume and Acuity, the next broad stroke in provider evaluation is these high level Outcomes. Note that although LOS is an Outcome, it is grouped within the Efficiency category.	Patient Care
Efficiency	Length of Stay, Acuity Adjusted Cost, Readmission Rates	Given Volumes and Outcomes, are they achieved with appropriate use of resources? Readmission is included here because a readmission can be viewed as "re-work."	Systems-Based Practice
Processes of Care	Core Measures and Compliance with Other Best Practices; May Include Drug and Blood Utilization	As we drill down into the details of patient care, we get to individual Processes, which, if performed well, are assumed to lead to better Outcomes. Providers with good Outcomes should also have higher scores on valid Process measures.	Patient Care

TQ CATEGORY	MEASURE SUMMARY	RATIONALE	ACGME CATEGORY
Privilege 1: Upper Endoscopy (example)	Volume, Acuity, Processes; Outcomes and Efficiency Measures Clustered by Specific Privileges	This approach clusters all the key metrics by privilege, especially helpful for Surgeons and Interventionalists. Grouping these metrics together provides clearer view of the provider's performance by Privilege, tracked over time, and compared to peers.	Patient Care, Systems-Based Practice
Privilege 2	Volume, Acuity, Processes, Outcomes, and Efficiency Measures Clustered by Specific Privileges	Create enough categories to cover the provider's main privileges.	Patient Care, Systems-Based Practice
Patient Satisfaction	Results of Patient Satisfaction Surveys and Validated Patient Complaints	Important metrics that reflect the patients' perceptions of their care are placed in a specific category.	Interpersonal and Communication Skills
Citizenship	Timely Completion of Medical Records, Including Discharge Summaries, Operative Notes, and History/Physicals. Compliance with Medical Staff Bylaws, Rules, and Regulations; Internal Staff Surveys and/or Validated Complaints. Participation in Medical Staff Committees and teaching for residency programs; .CME Credits per Quarter.	In addition to performance in Patient Care, how the provider works within the organization and with his/her peers is important, and bundled in this category. CME is added here on the assumption that staying current with continuing education is part of each provider's obligation to the care community.	Professionalism, Medical Knowledge
Review	Count of all Cases Peer Reviewed, with Outcomes of Reviews. Risk Management Claims Pending and Settled. Review of Any Issues, including Invasive Procedure, Infection Control, Blood Usage, P and T, etc.	Reviews are listed separately, even though they will cover cases that have been summarized above.	Practice-Based Learning and Improvement

37

Table 1.3 List of Possible Profiles for Large Multi-Specialty Hospital (count the x's, not the rows)

SPECIALTY	MD/DO/DPM/DDS	APC
Anesthesia	x	x
Surgery: General (to include Colon/Rectal, Plastics)	x	x
Bariatric surgery	x	
Urology	x	
CV, Vasc, and Thoracic Surgery	x	
Trauma/Acute Surgery	x	x
Otolaryngology	x	
Ophthalmology	x	
Orthopedics	x	x
Podiatry	x	
Neurosurgery	x	x
Oral/Dental Surgery	x	
Dentistry (Adult and Pediatric)	x	
Gynecology (Not OB)	x	
Gynecology Oncology	x	
OB and Gyn	x	x
Obstetrics	x	
Wound Care/Hyperbarics	x	
Hospitalist Medicine	x	x
Internal Medicine	x	x
Family Medicine (Incl Ped and OB with Correct Peer Groups)	x	x
Endocrinology/Diabetes Care	x	x
Intensivists (May Include Pulmonary/Anesthesia)	x	x
Interventional Cardiology	x	
Cardiology	x	
Gastroenterology	x	x
Pulmonary Medicine (Not Intensivists)	x	
Sleep Medicine	x	
Nephrology	x	x
Neurology	x	
Tele-Neurology	x	
Hematology and Oncology	x	x
Pediatrics	x	x

SPECIALTY	MD/DO/DPM/DDS	APC
Neonatology	X	X
Rehabilitation	X	
Pain Management	X	
Psychiatry	X	
Tele-Psychiatry	X	
Hospice and Palliative care	X	
Emergency Medicine	X	X
Pathology - (Excel)	X	
Radiology	X	X
Radiation Oncology	X	
Interventional Radiology	X	
Tele-Radiology	X	
Consulting (All Low Volume Consultants)	X	X

NOTES

NOTES

Chapter 2

Planning the First Meal: The Generic Profile

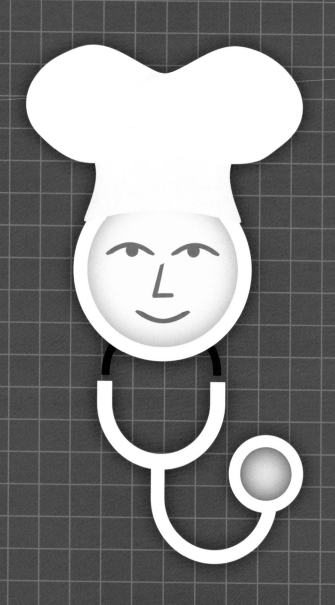

Planning the First Meal...

Let's go ahead and plan for our first meal – a balanced offering sure to delight all diners, surveyors, and providers alike. We'll start with the regular items that all providers with privileges need regardless of specialty, giving us a basis on which to build more exotic dishes in the future. As we add menu items, we will probably need to make additions to our shopping list, but before we leave the house with our shopping bags, we'll be sure to read Chapter 6 where we review the skills that every savvy shopper needs!

For our first profile, we want to create a generic foundation of the basics that apply to all providers with privileges. We'll then build on this as we branch into specialties and focus on privilege-based profiles. Using the third format, Talis Qualis (TQ) presented in Chapter 1, page 36, a Generic Profile might look like Table 2.1. Each category is described below with a discussion of the measures in this first Generic Profile.

We start with Volume as Attending, Consultant, and Procedure Provider, both as Principal Procedure Provider (the provider who did the principal procedure for each encounter), and any Procedure Provider (the provider who did any "secondary" procedures that follow the primary procedure). For example, consider an Upper Endoscopy done post-op for GI bleeding in a patient admitted for Surgical Hip Replacement; the Endoscopy would be a secondary procedure, with Hip Replacement as the principal procedure. If the data is available, it is best to categorize the Volume by Care Location: Inpatient, Outpatient, or Short Stay. Acuity will vary by Location, and these Volume numbers can be used as denominators for calculation of Length of Stay or other Efficiency measures.

For hospital inpatient measures, it is important to consider the characteristics of the patient population when creating indicators such as Length of Stay and Mortality Rate. For example, an average community hospital with 200-400 beds most likely provides services of Obstetrics, Pediatrics (including newborns), Medicine (including medical specialties and ICU), and Surgical Services (including surgical subspecialties and ICU) with or without a trauma service). In addition, it likely has inpatient Rehabilitation beds, Behavioral Health beds, and possibly Licensed Hospice beds.

The Average Length of Stay (ALOS) and Mortality Rate vary widely among these groups, making the distribution of services alone a determinate of the hospital's overall ALOS and Mortality Rate. For instance, consider this: a community hospital with 300 licensed beds may have a total of 19,000 annual discharges, including 3,000 deliveries and 3,000 healthy neonates, along with 100 Rehabilitation patients, and 400 Behavioral Health inpatient discharges, as well as 50 Licensed Hospice beds. The hospital ALOS may be 3.8 days for the 19,000 total discharges. However, if we remove OB/Neonatal (high Volume, low ALOS), the facility is left with 13,000 discharges with an ALOS of 4.3, a half day higher without the high Volume low ALOS services. It is easy to see that the overall ALOS can vary from year to year simply by changes in the Volume of the OB Service.

You may find it helpful to define subpopulations of similar services, to create a more homogeneous comparative population, both for external comparisons and for internal period-to-period comparisons. One means of accomplishing this would be to define 2 reporting populations for hospital indicators, including ALOS and Mortality:

1. All Inpatients: All discharges
2. Medical/Surgical Inpatients: All discharges minus discharges for Obstetrics, Newborns, Behavioral Health, Rehabilitation, and any Licensed Hospice beds

You may also want to create separate populations for large subspecialties, depending on the Case Mix at your hospital. The sample profiles provided in this volume will suggest metrics based on All Inpatients and Medical/Surgical Inpatients, as defined above.

Some measurement of the Severity of Illness of the provider's population is important. In referencing Severity, we mean how "sick" the patient is, as measured by the amount of resources required to get him/her to discharge. Severity correlates with Length of Stay, but that is not the only measure of Resource Use; most Severity models take into account the services administered during the stay, including Laboratory, Pharmacy, and Operating

Room costs, as well as the total number of days.

In many cases, the simplest initial approach to Severity Adjustment is to use the MS-DRG Relative Weights, which are used to determine hospital reimbursement per case. Each encounter assigned an MS-DRG has an associated Relative Weight (RW), which, when multiplied by the hospital's base reimbursement rate, determines its payment from Medicare. For a provider's patient population, these RWs can be averaged to produce a measure of the level of Severity, or Acuity, of the patient population. This is also known as Case Mix Index. One caution: MS-DRGs have been created strictly for reimbursement by Medicare, and do not cover pediatric diagnoses or common conditions in patients younger than 65 years of age.

There are a number of more sophisticated Severity Adjustment systems, including 3M's APR-DRGs. Note that APR-DRGs are "All-Patient" and cover procedures and conditions across the age continuum, including neonates and pediatrics. For each clinically coherent APR-DRG, there are 4 sub-classes each for Severity of Illness and Risk of Mortality. Recently, 3M has expanded its methodology to include Potentially Preventable Readmissions and Potentially Preventable Complications ("3M Health Information Systems," 2014). Indicators associated with these metrics may be of benefit as appropriate.

After Volume and Acuity, examine Outcomes of Care, the broadest being Mortality. Although controversial in the past, there is general agreement that adjusted Mortality Rates are reflective of quality (Berwick, Calkins, McCannon, & Hackbarth, 2006). In our Generic Profile, we include Mortality Counts, Number of Deaths/Time Period, and Rates, by Attending and Principal Procedure Provider, for all patient encounters as well as the Medical/Surgical subset.

In addition to Mortality, our TQ model includes measures of Complications of Care and Rare Events, as Attending and Principal Procedure Provider.

Traditionally, Complications of Care have been difficult to measure, requiring either voluntary reporting (as in traditional Surgical Morbidity and Mortality rounds), or screening measures, such as Counts of Returns to the Operating Room. However, many Medical Staff groups see the merit of including these measures in provider profiles.

One of the simplest approaches to measuring Complications is to use administrative data, which is generated at discharge when the patient's medical record is abstracted and coded. In 1994, the Agency for Healthcare

Research and Quality (AHRQ) created a set of quality measures that used hospital administrative data provided by the Healthcare Cost and Utilization Project (HCUP). These HCUP quality indicators took advantage of readily available administrative data to identify potential quality of care problems. In 1998, researchers at UCSF and the Stanford University Evidence-Based Practice Center reviewed and revised the original set of measures to create the AHRQ QIs (Quality Indicators), originally provided in 2 modules, Prevention Quality Indicators (PQIs) and Inpatient Quality Indicators (IQIs). By 2006, additional modules were added, Patient Safety Indicators (PSIs) and Pediatric Quality Indicators (PDIs) (Hughes, 2008).

Of the 4 AHRQ QI modules, the IQIs, PSIs, and PDIs are viewed as the most applicable to measuring inpatient Quality and Complications of Care; see Tables 2.2, 2.3, 2.4. A note of caution: these indicators are extensive; the PSIs in particular require complicated algorithms. AHRQ provides software for calculating the indicators; alternatively, the values can be obtained through IT vendors that provide comparative data packages.

Using administrative data by itself can be helpful in the search for Complications. In addition to patient demographics, the record contains the principal diagnosis, or the diagnosis which, after testing and treatment, is determined to be the primary reason for admission. Following the principal diagnosis are all the secondary diagnoses, followed by the principal and secondary procedures. In the ICD-9 CM system (in use as of this publication date), there are specific codes for Complications, with a section titled Injury and Poisoning, including codes ICD-9 800-999. However, it is often difficult to determine when the Injury or Complication occurred, and if any given Injury or Complication occurred as a result of treatment.[1]

For example, here are a series of codes for amputation complications:

ICD-9 997.60   Unspecified late complication of amputation stump
ICD-9 997.61   Neuroma of amputation stump
ICD-9 997.62   Infection (chronic) of amputation stump
ICD-9 997.69   Other amputation stump complication

---

[1]The United States will be converting to ICD-10 as of October 15, 2015, as of this publication date. During this transition period, we are providing examples of complications using the ICD-9 codes as illustrations, understanding that these will change in late 2015.

Most of these Complications are likely chronic, and not the result of care during the admission for which they are coded, making them less likely to be helpful for provider profiles. However, this administrative data became more useful in 2007, when a provision of the Deficit Reduction Act of 2005 (DRA) required that all secondary diagnoses be flagged to indicate if they were present on admission or not present on admission (POA/NPOA) ("Hospital-acquired conditions," 2014). At that time, POA/NPOA flags also became incorporated in the revised Universal Billing Form UB-04. This additional flag expanded the list of potential Complications beyond the 800-999 codes. For example, consider ICD-9 427.5, Cardiac Arrest. With the addition of the POA/NPOA flag, we can find patients who arrested during their hospital stays, versus those arriving in Cardiac Arrest.

Starting in October 2007, the DRA required that the Secretary of the US Department of Health and Human Services begin to identify conditions that were high cost, high Volume, or both. This identification resulted in the assignment of a case to an MS-DRG with a higher payment when present as a secondary diagnosis, and could reasonably have been prevented through the application of evidence-based guidelines. For discharges after October 1, 2007, Medicare prospective payment hospitals do not receive the higher payment for cases when a selected condition was acquired during hospitalization. Instead, the case is paid as though the secondary diagnosis is not present. These specified conditions are designated Hospital Acquired Conditions, or HACs ("Hospital-acquired conditions," 2014). A list of HAC categories in the CMS HAC payment provision for Fiscal Years 2014 and 2015 is provided in Table 2.5.

The POA/NPOA flag on diagnoses can be helpful in finding potential Complications, whether they be CMS designated HACs, or conditions determined by your Medical Staff; these might include those that are unique to your hospital, location, or patient population. In either case, the Complication should be avoidable during the course of the patient's care, and attributable to a provider.

Even when a Complication is identified as a preventable consequence of care, it is often difficult to attribute it to a single provider. The closest attribution is to the Principal Procedure Provider for elective surgical cases. Further, those with experience understand that attribution is even harder for complex medical cases with long hospital stays. In reality, there is no established means of assuring proper attribution. As you address these indicators, it is important to keep in mind the complexity associated with Complication measures and their attribution. Your hospital's Medical Staff may establish protocols for standard attribution in order to ensure consistency in determining responsibility; once such protocols are established, they may be used as rationale or as a guide for situations when attribution is unclear within the medical record.

Finally, it can be helpful to examine the Outcomes of the patients with Complications; for example, consider the Mortality Rate for all patients with a diagnosis of Myocardial Infarction or Pneumonia NPOA. Death after a Complication may be seen as a "failure to rescue," and can therefore be viewed as an important aspect of performance. A recent study of Cardiac Surgery Outcomes from a 33 center quality collaborative indicated that although hospitals may have similar Complication Rates associated with Cardiac Surgery, some are better at treating Complications ("rescue"), lowering the Risk of Mortality (Reddy et al., 2013). Additional research supports the argument that high performance includes both minimizing the Risk of Complications at the outset, and recognizing and treating them effectively when they occur.

Once we have Volume/Acuity and Outcomes, the next set of measures address Efficiency, how well are resources used to restore the patient's health to a stage compatible with discharge. Here we see Average Length of Stay by Attending and Principal Procedure Provider, Adjusted and Unadjusted, for all discharges, and for just the Medical/Surgical population. Note that we have included here Readmissions and Returns to Surgery by provider type, on the assumption that both are a form of re-work, increasing the total resource use and cost.

If your hospital has a calculation for Cost per Discharge, that Cost can be divided by the MS-DRG RW, or the weights associated with APR-DRG Severity levels, to create a Cost/Relative Weight. Since these weights are used for reimbursement, the ratio is a general index of Efficiency of Care.

Next come measures for Processes of Care, which ideally correlate with Outcomes. This is a good place to put the TJC and CMS Core Measures, now known as: The Joint Commission Measures; Hospital Inpatient Quality Reporting Program measures (HIQR); and Hospital Outpatient Quality Reporting Program measures (HOQR). These measure sets focus primarily on measuring Processes of Care, and are readily available due to their associated reporting requirements. See Table 2.6 for a list of these measures which are active in 2015. As always, look for measures with accurate provider attribution, which reflect performance in key areas of patient care.

At this point, we have a pretty good picture of the provider's activity and performance, including Mortality, Complications, and Length of Stay, along with measures of Efficiency and Processes of Care. Next, we turn to the patients themselves for survey-based Patient Satisfaction measures and any validated Patient Complaints.

Moving along, we encounter the broad category of Citizenship, which includes Timely Completion of Histories and Physicals, Operative Notes, and Discharge Summaries, as well as Compliance with Medical Staff Rules and Regulations. Including measures of Staff Satisfaction is helpful; these are ideally based on periodic surveys that are provider specific. CME Credits can be added here as well, as part of being a good hospital citizen is maintaining appropriate levels of certification and recent training.

The final category in this TQ Generic Profile addresses any cases that have been reviewed as part of the Medical Staff Peer Review process, or other Reviews. At your discretion, metrics associated with Claims data may also be included here.

Our proposed TQ Generic Profile is designed to cover the basics of all providers with privileges, regardless of specialty. In our experience, starting here is logical, but is not as easy as it might first appear. Most of the major issues with provider profiling will be encountered in this first Generic Profile. Pay close attention to the following associated tasks:

- Define the denominator populations carefully and ensure they are the same for the provider's measure and for any comparison data.
- Adjust for Severity and Risk of Mortality as well as possible. MS-DRG RWs can be used as a back-up, but CMS provides no Risk of Mortality adjustment. Consider a commercial Risk Adjustment program to meet this demand.
- Pick Complication measures carefully and sparingly at the outset. There continues to be discussion of how these measures truly measure Avoidable Complications, and to whom they should be attributed.

Overuse of Complication measures may become a distraction during the process of adopting profiles by the Medical Staff. See Chapter 7 for more on implementation and adoption. Realize that Attending attribution—and, in truth, attribution identification as a whole—is always an issue; it is one that is best approached directly by the Medical Staff in its bylaws, rules, and regulations.

- A good cost-accounting system will help you construct good Efficiency measures. See Chapter 6 for more detail.
- You will need access to your Core Measures, and provider-specific Patient Satisfaction data.
- Internal Staff satisfaction surveys are helpful.
- Updated, robust Medical Staff bylaws, rules, and regulations are essential, especially in relation to the OPPE, FPPE, and Peer Review processes.

A Step Beyond Generic: Medical and Surgical Procedural Profiles

In Chapter 1, we outlined the number of profiles a hospital likely needs, and the order in which these might be built. Recall that we started with the Generic Profile, as outlined above, which covers basic performance for all members of the Medial Staff with privileges who admit and discharge patients. We then added the 4 specialties that generally function outside the admission/discharge patient model: Pathology, Radiology, Emergency Medicine, and Anesthesiology. These will be covered in Chapter 4.

The next step is to expand the Generic Profile to better cover the performance of the 2 major groups among the Medical Staff: those who primarily perform procedures (such as surgery and interventional procedures), and those who provide day-to-day bedside care, such as Internists, Hospitalists, Pediatricians, and Intensivists. The TQ Generic Profile, outlined above, covers both groups appropriately for Volume, Acuity, Efficiency, Patient Satisfaction, Citizenship, and Review. The categories where measures can be added to support these 2 groups are Clinical Outcomes and Processes of Care.

A provider profile tailored to Surgeons/Proceduralists might include some of the following Outcome and Process measures added to the Generic Profile:

Outcomes:
- Unscheduled Returns to the Operating Room Following an Elective Procedure
- Principal Procedure Provider, Medical/Surgical, Percent Readmitted within 30 Days
- AHRQ IQI 90 Inpatient Quality Composite, Procedures Mortality
- Foreign Body Left During a Procedure
- Intraoperative Injuries
- Postoperative Hematoma
- Postoperative Shock

Processes of Care:
- Selected Core Measures: See Table 2.6
- Appropriate Use of Blood and Blood Products
- Late OR Starts
- Call Availability

A provider profile for Internists/Hospitalists/Family Medicine practitioners might include some of the following Outcome and Process measures added to the TQ Generic Profile:

Outcomes:
- Acute MI, Mortality Rate
- AHRQ IQI 91 Inpatient Quality Composite, Conditions Mortality
- Iatrogenic Pneumothorax with Venous Catheter – Per 1000 Inpatients
- Severe Sepsis or Septic Shock – Mortality Rate
- COPD – Percent Readmit within 30 Days
- COPD – Mortality Rate

Processes of Care:
- Poor Glycemic Control – Per 1000 Inpatients
- Selected Core Measures: See Table 2.6

- Use of Drugs
  - o Drug Utilization by Diagnosis
    - Acute Myocardial Infarction
    - Pneumonia
  - o Antibiotic Use by Diagnosis
    - Pneumonia
    - Diverticulitis

Summary

In this chapter, we have demonstrated how to build a Generic Profile that covers the basic measures that apply to all providers with privileges. We have built a sample profile in the TQ format, with mapping of domains to the ACGME format, including measures for Volume and Acuity, Clinical Outcomes with Mortality and Complications, Efficiency with Length of Stay and Readmissions, as well as Processes of Care, Patient Satisfaction, Citizenship, and Review by Peers. We have also shown how this base profile can be extended to better cover Surgical/Procedural and Medical providers by adding additional measures.

In Chapter 3, we will examine how to add privilege-based measures to our Generic Profile, with Chapter 4 devoted to creating profiles for the 4 major specialties that are difficult to cover with administrative discharge data: Pathology, Radiology, Emergency Medicine, and Anesthesiology.

Reference List:

"3M Health Information Systems: Classification and grouping." (2014). Retrieved from http://solutions.3m.com/wps/portal/3M/en_US/Health-Information-Systems/HIS/Products-and-Services/Classification-and-Grouping/

Berwick D.M., Calkins D.R., McCannon, D.J., & Hackbarth, A.D. (2006). The 100,000 lives campaign: Setting a goal and a deadline for improving health care quality. *The Journal of the American Medical Association* (295), 324-327.

"Hospital-acquired conditions and present on admission indicator reporting provision." (2014). Medicare Learning Network, Centers for Medicare & Medicaid Services, September 2014. Retrieved from http://www.cms.gov/Outreach-and-Education/Medicare-Learning-Network-MLN/MLNProducts/Downloads/wPOAFactSheet.pdf

Hughes, R.G., Ed. (2008). *Patient Safety and Quality: An Evidence-Based Handbook for Nurses.* Rockville, MD: Agency for Healthcare Research and Quality. Retrieved from http://www.ncbi.nlm.nih.gov/books/NBK2651/

"Inpatient quality indicators technical specifications – Version 4.5." (2013). AHRQ. Retrieved from http://www.qualityindicators.ahrq.gov/Modules/IQI_TechSpec.aspx

"Patient safety indicators technical specifications updates – Version 4.5a." (2014). AHRQ. Retrieved from http://www.qualityindicators.ahrq.gov/Modules/PSI_TechSpec.aspx

"Pediatric quality indicators technical specifications – Version 4.5." (2013). AHRQ. Retrieved from http://www.qualityindicators.ahrq.gov/Modules/PDI_TechSpec.aspx

Reddy, H.G., Shih, T., Englesbe, M.J., Shannon, F.L., Theurer, P.F., Herbert, M., & Prager, R.L. (2013). Analyzing failure to rescue: Is this an opportunity for outcome improvement in cardiac surgery? *The Society of Thoracic Surgeons,* (95): 1976-81.

Table 2.1 Generic Provider Profile

CATEGORY	MEASURE	ACGME
Volume		
	Volume as Attending: All Patients	Patient Care
	Volume as Attending: Medical/Surgical	Patient Care
	Volume as Attending Outpatient/Short Stay	Patient Care
	Volume as Consultant: Total Inpatients Seen in Consultation	Patient Care
	Volume as Consultant: Medical/Surgical	Patient Care
	Volume of Outpatient Procedures/Short Stay	Patient Care
	Volume: Total Procedures Performed, Inpatient and Outpatient	Patient Care
	Volume as Principal Procedure Provider: Medical/Surgical	Patient Care
	Volume of Procedures as Any Procedure Provider, Medical/Surgical	Patient Care
Acuity		
	CMI as Attending: Medical/Surgical	Patient Care
	Average CMI as Principle Procedure Provider, Medical/Surgical	Patient Care
Clinical Outcome		
	Mortality Rate Risk Adjusted as Attending, Medical/Surgical	Patient Care
	Mortality Count as Attending, Medical/Surgical	Patient Care
	Mortality Rate Risk Adjusted as Principal Procedure Provider, Medical/Surgical	Patient Care
	Mortality Count as Principal Procedure Provider, Medical/Surgical	Patient Care
	Mortality following a Procedure, as Principal Procedure Provider, Medical/Surgical, (Rare Event)	Patient Care
	Mortality Rate of Pts w/ Major Complications as Attending	Patient Care
	Mortality Rate of Pts w/ Major Complications as Principal Procedure Provider	Patient Care
	Complications of Care, as Attending, Medical/Surgical	Patient Care
	Complications of Care, as Principal Procedure Provider, Medical/Surgical	Patient Care
	Rare Events as Attending, Medical/Surgical	Patient Care
	Rare Events as Principal Procedure Provider, Medical/Surgical	Patient Care

CATEGORY	MEASURE	ACGME
Efficiency		
	Average LOS as Attending, All Patients	Systems-Based Practice
	Average LOS as Attending, Medical/Surgical	Systems-Based Practice
	Average LOS as Principal Procedure Provider, All Patients	Systems-Based Practice
	Average LOS as Principal Procedure Provider, Medical/Surgical	Systems-Based Practice
	% Readmission within 30 Days as Attending, All Patients	Systems-Based Practice
	% Readmission within 30 Days as Attending, Medical/Surgical	Systems-Based Practice
	% Readmission within 30 Days as Principal Procedure Provider, All Inpatients	Systems-Based Practice
	% Readmission within 30 Days as Principal Procedure Provider, Medical/Surgical	Systems-Based Practice
	% Return to Surgery as Principal Procedure Provider, Medical/Surgical	Systems-Based Practice
	Cost/Relative Weight as Attending, All Patients	Systems-Based Practice
	Cost/Relative Weight as Attending, Medical/Surgical	Systems-Based Practice
	Cost/Relative Weight as Principal Procedure Provider, All Patients	Systems-Based Practice
	Cost/Relative Weight as Principal Procedure Provider, Medical/Surgical	Systems-Based Practice
Processes of Care		
	Core Measures - AMI, CHF, SCIP, PN, STK, VTE, etc.	Patient Care
	Appropriate Use of Blood and Blood Products	Patient Care
	Other	Patient Care
	Validated Patient Complaints	Interpersonal and Communication skills
	Patient Satisfaction – Survey-Based [Hospital Vendor or HCAHPS, Provider Communication]	Interpersonal and Communication Skills

continued >>

Table 2.1 *continued....*

CATEGORY	MEASURE	ACGME
Patient Satisfaction		
	Validated Patient Complaints	Interpersonal and Communication skills
	Patient Satisfaction – Survey-Based [Hospital Vendor or HCAHPS, Provider Communication]	Interpersonal and Communication skills
Citizenship		
	Timely Completion of Histories and Physicals	Professionalism
	Timely Completion of Operative Notes	Professionalism
	Timely Completion of Discharge Summaries	Professionalism
	Validated Noncompliance with Medical Staff Rules and Regulations	Professionalism
	Staff Satisfaction: Relationships with Physicians, Communication and Responsiveness	Professionalism
	CME Credits per Quarter	Medical Knowledge
Review		
	Total Peer Cases Reviewed	Practice-Based Learning and Improvement
	Total Cases: Care Excellent	Practice-Based Learning and Improvement
	Total Cases: Appropriate Care	Practice-Based Learning and Improvement
	Total Cases: Opportunity for Improvement	Practice-Based Learning and Improvement
	Total Cases: System Opportunity for Improvement	Practice-Based Learning and Improvement
	Totals Pending Claims	Practice-Based Learning and Improvement
	Claims Settled	Practice-Based Learning and Improvement
	Pending Judgments	Practice-Based Learning and Improvement

CATEGORY	MEASURE	ACGME
Review, continued...		
	Invasive Procedure Issue (Review Validated)	Practice-Based Learning and Improvement
	Infection Control Issue (Review Validated)	Practice-Based Learning and Improvement
	Blood Usage Issue (Review Validated)	Practice-Based Learning and Improvement
	Pharmacy and Therapeutics (Review Validated)	Practice-Based Learning and Improvement
	Conscious Sedation Issue (Review Validated)	Practice-Based Learning and Improvement
	Restraint Issue (Review Validated)	Practice-Based Learning and Improvement
	Inappropriate Behavior (Review Validated)	Practice-Based Learning and Improvement
	Patient Compliant (Review Validated)	Practice-Based Learning and Improvement

Table 2.2 AHRQ Inpatient Quality Indicators

IQI 01	Esophageal Resection Volume
IQI 02	Pancreatic Resection Volume
IQI 04	Abdominal Aortic Aneurysm (AAA) Repair Volume
IQI 05	Coronary Artery Bypass Graft (CABG) Volume
IQI 06	Percutaneous Coronary Intervention (PCI) Volume
IQI 07	Carotid Endarterectomy Volume
IQI 08	Esophageal Resection Mortality Rate
IQI 09	Pancreatic Resection Mortality Rate
IQI 11	Abdominal Aortic Aneurysm (AAA) Repair Mortality Rate
IQI 12	Coronary Artery Bypass Graft (CABG) Mortality Rate
IQI 13	Craniotomy Mortality Rate
IQI 14	Hip Replacement Mortality Rate
IQI 15	Acute Myocardial Infarction (AMI) Mortality Rate
IQI 16	Heart Failure Mortality Rate
IQI 17	Acute Stroke Mortality Rate
IQI 18	Gastrointestinal Hemorrhage Mortality Rate
IQI 19	Hip Fracture Mortality Rate
IQI 20	Pneumonia Mortality Rate
IQI 21	Cesarean Delivery Rate, Uncomplicated
IQI 22	Vaginal Birth After Cesarean (VBAC) Delivery Rate, Uncomplicated
IQI 23	Laparoscopic Cholecystectomy Rate
IQI 24	Incidental Appendectomy in the Elderly Rate
IQI 25	Bilateral Cardiac Catheterization Rate
IQI 26	Coronary Artery Bypass Graft (CABG) Rate
IQI 27	Percutaneous Coronary Intervention (PCI) Rate
IQI 28	Hysterectomy Rate
IQI 29	Laminectomy or Spinal Fusion Rate
IQI 30	Percutaneous Coronary Intervention (PCI) Mortality Rate
IQI 31	Carotid Endarterectomy Mortality Rate
IQI 32	Acute Myocardial Infarction (AMI) Mortality Rate, Without Transfer Cases
IQI 33	Primary Cesarean Delivery Rate, Uncomplicated
IQI 34	Vaginal Birth After Cesarean (VBAC) Rate, All
IQI 90	Mortality for Selected Procedures: IQI 9, 11, 12, 13, 14, 30, 31.
IQI 91	Mortality for Selected Conditions: IQI 15, 16, 17, 18, 19, 20.

("Inpatient quality indicators technical specifications – Version 4.5," 2013)

Table 2.3 AHRQ Patient Safety Indicators

PSI 02	Death Rate in Low-Mortality Diagnosis Related Groups (DRGs)
PSI 03	Pressure Ulcer Rate
PSI 04	Death Rate among Surgical Inpatients with Serious Treatable Conditions
PSI 05	Retained Surgical Item or Unretrieved Device Fragment Count
PSI 06	Iatrogenic Pneumothorax Rate
PSI 07	Central Venous Catheter-Related Blood Stream Infection Rate
PSI 08	Postoperative Hip Fracture Rate
PSI 09	Perioperative Hemorrhage or Hematoma Rate
PSI 10	Postoperative Physiologic and Metabolic Derangement Rate
PSI 11	Postoperative Respiratory Failure Rate
PSI 12	Perioperative Pulmonary Embolism or Deep Vein Thrombosis Rate
PSI 13	Postoperative Sepsis Rate
PSI 14	Postoperative Wound Dehiscence Rate
PSI 15	Accidental Puncture or Laceration Rate
PSI 16	Transfusion Reaction Count
PSI 19	Obstetric Trauma Rate-Vaginal Delivery without Instrument
PSI 21	Retained Surgical Item or Unretrieved Device Fragment Rate
PSI 22	Iatrogenic Pneumothorax Rate
PSI 23	Central Venous Catheter-Related Blood Stream Infection Rate
PSI 24	Postoperative Wound Dehiscence Rate
PSI 25	Accidental Puncture or Laceration Rate
PSI 26	Transfusion Reaction Rate
PSI 27	Postoperative Hemorrhage or Hematoma Rate
PSI 90	Patient Safety for Selected Indicators: PSI 3, 6, 7, 8, 9, 10, 11, 12, 13, 14, 15

("Patient quality indicators technical specifications – Version 4.5," 2013)

Table 2.4 AHRQ Pediatric Quality Indicators

NQI 01	Neonatal Iatrogenic Pneumothorax Rate
NQI 02	Neonatal Mortality Rate
NQI 03	Neonatal Blood Stream Infection Rate
PDI 01	Accidental Puncture or Laceration Rate
PDI 02	Pressure Ulcer Rate
PDI 03	Retained Surgical Item or Unretrieved Device Fragment Count
PDI 05	Iatrogenic Pneumothorax Rate
PDI 06	RACHS-1 Pediatric Heart Surgery Mortality Rate
PDI 07	RACHS-1 Pediatric Heart Surgery Volume
PDI 08	Perioperative Hemorrhage or Hematoma Rate
PDI 09	Postoperative Respiratory Failure Rate
PDI 10	Postoperative Sepsis Rate
PDI 11	Postoperative Wound Dehiscence Rate
PDI 12	Central Venous Catheter-Related Blood Stream Infection Rate
PDI 13	Transfusion Reaction Count
PDI 14	Asthma Admission Rate
PDI 15	Diabetes Short-term Complications Admission Rate
PDI 16	Gastroenteritis Admission Rate
PDI 17	Perforated Appendix Admission Rate
PDI 18	Urinary Tract Infection Admission Rate
PDI 19	Pediatric Safety for Selected Indicators: PDI 1, 2, 5, 8, 9, 10,1 1, 12
PDI 90	Pediatric Quality Overall Composite: PDI 14, 15, 16, 18.
PDI 91	Pediatric Quality Acute Composite: PDI 16, 18.
PDI 92	Pediatric Quality Chronic Composite: PDI 14, 15.

("Pediatric quality indicators technical specifications – Version 4.5," 2013)

Table 2.5 CMS HAC Categories for FY 2014 and 2015

Foreign Object Retained after Surgery	
Air Embolism	
Blood Incompatibility	
Pressure Ulcer Stages III & IV	
Falls and Trauma	
	Fracture
	Dislocation
	Intracranial Injury
	Crushing Injury
	Burn
	Other Injuries
Catheter-Associated Urinary Tract Infection (CAUTI)	
Vascular Catheter-Associated Infection	
Manifestation of Poor Glycemic Control	
	Diabetic Ketoacidosis
	Nonketotic Hyperosmolar Coma
	Hypoglycemic Coma
	Secondary Diabetes with Ketoacidosis
	Secondary Diabetes with Hyperosmolarity
Surgical Site Infection, Mediastinitis, following Coronary Artery Bypass Graft (CABG)	
Surgical Site Infection, following Certain Orthopedic Procedures	
	Spine
	Neck
	Shoulder
	Elbow
Surgical Site Infection following Bariatric Surgery for Obesity	
	Laparoscopic Gastric Bypass
	Gastroenterostomy
	Laparoscopic Gastric Restrictive Surgery
Surgical Site Infection following Cardiac Implantable Electronic Device (CIED)	
Deep Vein Thrombosis and Pulmonary Embolism following Certain Orthopedic Procedures	
	Total Knee Replacement
	Hip Replacement
Iatrogenic Pneumothorax with Venous Catheterization	

("Hospital-acquired conditions," 2014)

Table 2.6 Measure Table for Hospital IQR, IPFQR, Hospital OQR, and The Joint Commission *(Note: Current as of 1/15/2015; consult your Core Measure vendor specifications for more information).*

MEASURE	MEASURE NAME
AMI-7a	Fibrinolytic Therapy Received within 30 Minutes of Hospital Arrival
APEC	Assessment of Patient Experience of Care (FY2016 PD)
CAC-3	Home Management Plan of Care (HMPC) Document Given to Patient/Caregiver
Cost-AMI	AMI Payment per Episode of Care
Cost-HF	HF Payment per Episode of Care
Cost -MSPB	Medicare Spending per Beneficiary
Cost-PN	PN Payment per Episode of Care
ED-1	Median Time from ED Arrival to ED Departure for Admitted ED Patients
ED-2	Admit Decision Time to ED Departure Time for Admitted Patients
EHR	Use of an Electronic Health Record (FY2016PD)
FUH	Follow-up After Hospitalization
HAI	Central Line Associated Bloodstream Infection (CLABSI)
HAI	Surgical Site Infection (Colon / Hysterectomy)
HAI	Catheter-Associated Urinary Tract Infection (CAUTI)
HAI	MRSA Bacteremia
HAI	Clostridium Difficile (CDI)
HAI	Healthcare Personnel Influenza Vaccination (2015-2016 flu season)
HBIPS-1	Admission Screening for Violence Risk, Substance Use, Psychological Trauma History and Patient Strengths completed
HBIPS-2	Hours of Physical Restraint Use
HBIPS-3	Hours of Seclusion Use
HBIPS-4	Patients Discharged on Multiple Antipsychotic Meds
HBIPS-5	Patients Discharged on Multiple Antipsychotic Medications with Appropriate Justification
HBIPS-6	Post Discharge Continuing Care Plan Created
HBIPS-7	Post Discharge Continuing Care Plan Transmitted to Next level of Care Provider Upon Discharge
HCAHPS	HCAHPS Survey
HCP Influenza Vaccination	Influenza Vaccination Coverage Among Health Care Personnel (2015-2016 flu season)
IMM-2	Influenza Immunization (FY2017 PD)
Mort-30-AMI	Acute Myocardial Infarction (AMI) 30-day Mortality Rate
Mort-30-HF	Heart Failure (HF) 30-day Mortality Rate

MEASURE	MEASURE NAME
Mort-30-PN	Pneumonia (PN) 30-day Mortality Rate
Mort-CABG	CABG Surgery 30-day All-Cause Risk-Standardized Mortality Rate
Mort-COPD	COPD 30-day Mortality Rate
Mort-STK	Stroke 30-day Mortality Rate
OP-1	Median Time to Fibrinolysis
OP-2	Fibrinolytic Therapy Received within 30 Minutes
OP-3	Median Time to Transfer to Another Facility for Acute Coronary Intervention
OP-4	Aspirin at Arrival
OP-5	Median Time to ECG
OP-8	MRI Lumbar Spine for Low Back Pain
OP-9	Mammography Follow-up Rates
OP-10	Abdomen CT - Use of Contrast Material
OP-11	Thorax CT - Use of Contrast Material
OP-12	The Ability for Providers w/ HIT to Receive Lab Data Electronically Directly into their ONC Certified EHR System as Discrete Searchable Data
OP-13	Cardiac Imaging for Preoperative Risk Assessment for Non Cardiac Low Risk Surgery
OP-14	Simultaneous Use of Brain Computed Tomography (CT) and Sinus Computed Tomography (CT)
OP-15	Use of Brain Computed Tomography (CT) in the Emergency Department for Atraumatic Headache
OP-17	Tracking Clinical Results Between Visits
OP-18	Median Time from ED Arrival to ED Departure for Discharged ED Patients
OP-20	Door to Diagnostic Evaluation by a Qualified Medical Personnel
OP-21	Median Time to Pain Mgt. for Long Bone Fracture
OP-22	Left Without Being Seen
OP-23	Head CT or MRI Scan Results for Acute Ischemic Stroke or Hemorrhagic Stroke Patients who Received Head CT or MRI Scan Interpretation Within 45 minutes of ED Arrival
OP-25	Safe Surgery Checklist
OP-26	Hospital OP Vol. on Selected OP Surg. Procedure
OP-27	Influenza Vaccination Coverage among Healthcare Personnel (2015-2016 flu season)
OP-29	Endoscopy/Polyp Surveillance: Appropriate Follow-up Interval for Normal Colonoscopy in Average Risk Patients

continued >>

Table 2.6 *continued...*

MEASURE	MEASURE NAME
OP-30	Endoscopy/Polyp surveillance: Colonoscopy Interval for Patients with a History of Adenomatous Polyps- Avoidance of Inappropriate Use
OP-31	Cataracts: Improvement in Patient's Visual Function within 90 days Following Cataract Surgery
OP-32	Facility 7-Day Risk-Standardized Hospital Visit Rate after Outpatient Colonoscopy
PC-01	Elective Delivery Prior to 39 Completed Weeks of Gestation
PC-02	Cesarean Section
PC-03	Antenatal Steroids
PC-04	Health Care-Assoc. Bloodstream Inf. in Newborns
PC-05	Exclusive Breast Milk Feeding
PC-05a	Mother's Initial Feeding Plan
PSI-4	Death Among Surgical Inpatients with Serious Treatable Complications
PSI-90 Composite	Complication/Patient Safety for Selected Indicators
Readm-30-AMI	AMI 30-day Risk Standardized
Readm-30-HF	Heart Failure (HF) 30-day Risk Standardized
Readm-30-HWR	Hospital-Wide All-Cause Unplanned Readmission (HWR)*
Readm-30-PN	Pneumonia (PN) 30-day Risk Standardized
Readm-30-TH/TKA	30-day Risk Standardized Readmission Following Total Hip/ Total Knee Arthroplasty
Readm-CABG	CABG 30-day Risk Standardized Readmission
Readm-COPD	COPD 30-day Risk Standardized Readmission
Readm-STK	Stroke 30-day Risk Standardized
Registry-GenSurg	Participation in a Systematic Clinical Database Registry for General Surgery
Registry-NSC	Participation in a Systematic Clinical Database Registry for Nursing Sensitive Care
Registry-SSCL	Safe Surgery Checklist Use
SEPSIS	Severe Sepsis and Septic Shock: Management Bundle
STK-1	VTE Prophylaxis
STK-2	Antithrombotic Therapy for Ischemic Stroke
STK-3	Anticoagulation Therapy for Afib/flutter
STK-4	Thrombolytic Therapy for Acute Ischemic Stroke
STK-5	Antithrombotic Therapy By End of Hospital Day 2
STK-6	Discharged on Statin
STK-8	Stroke Education
STK-10	Assessed for Rehab

MEASURE	MEASURE NAME
SUB-1	Alcohol Use Screening
SUB-2	Alcohol Use Brief Intervention Provided or Offered
SUB-3	Alcohol and Other Drug Use Disorder Treatment Provided or Offered at Discharge
Surgical Complicn	Hip/Knee Complication: Hospital-level Risk-Standardized Complication Rate (RSCR) Following Elective Primary Total Hip Arthroplasty
TOB-1	Tobacco Use Screening
TOB-2	Tobacco Use Treatment Provided or Offered
TOB-2a	Tobacco Use Treatment (FY2017PD)
TOB-3	Tobacco Use Treatment Provided or Offered at Discharge
VTE-1	VTE Prophylaxis
VTE-2	ICU VTE Prophylaxis
VTE-3	VTE Patients with Anticoagulation Overlap Therapy
VTE-5	VTE Discharge Instructions
VTE-6	Incidence of Potentially Preventable VTE

NOTES

NOTES

Chapter 3

Customizing the Menu: Privilege-Based Profiles

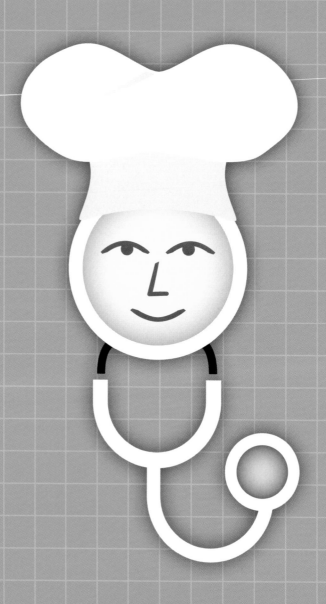

Time to Refine the Menus...

Now that you know that your customers are getting healthy fare and will not starve, ask yourself if they are really happy dining at your table. What may satisfy your customers early on may become tiring with time; it is quite likely that you will need to expand the offerings depending on their special tastes and needs.

The Joint Commission will ask for special items based on provider privileges, and, in turn, your providers will need this more specific information to improve their performance over time, both as individuals and as groups. Understanding your customers' needs is of great benefit here—so keep considering these as you move forward in your work.

It's really the time to be focused, and diligent. At the same time, don't forget to start slowly and carefully, but don't quit early – look for those extra items by specialty. We'll spend more time on shopping in Chapter 6.

At this point, since we have built the Generic Profile, we have all the basics for a provider with privileges, regardless of department or specialty. However, even if the most recent visit from an accreditation team did not include a focus on specific privilege-based measures, it will the next time. Now is the time to prepare.

All accrediting bodies want to see performance measured in the areas where each provider has privileges, regardless of the frequency required for measuring provider performance. This makes sense. If you or a member of your family presents to your local Emergency Room with chest pain and ST elevation on the EKG, you want to know that your Interventional Cardiologist is skilled at opening up occluded coronary arteries with high success rates, low morbidity, and low mortality. Only metrics that address these specific interventional privileges can illustrate these performance deliverables.

The quickest path toward privilege-based measures starts with your hospital's privileging system. A description of privileging systems is beyond the scope of this book, but details can be found in a number of recent publications ("Credentialing and privileging," 2014; "Hospital privileging," 2015). It is fair to say that the current trend is toward the core approach, whereby all providers who have completed training and board certification in a specialty are eligible for categories of privileges, with final approval based on demonstration of experience and acceptable performance. While TJC does not support a certain privileging methodology over another, it emphasizes that it is not acceptable to assume that all providers should be granted all privileges ("Core/bundled," 2008). Your hospital likely has an established means for ensuring even core, or basic privileges, are granted only to those providers who can perform the service or procedure.

Consider a situation in a hospital that uses core privileging, with a physician who has completed training in Gastroenterology and passed her boards may be considered eligible for certain privileges that are considered "core" based on her training. That is, all graduates of accredited Gastroenterology training programs are expected to have been trained and be able to demonstrate competency in certain basic techniques and procedures. Medical Staff bylaws, rules, and regulations provide guidance on how to ensure she is granted privileges she can, in fact, perform. There may be other, more advanced procedures that require additional training; these would be added as options to the core, for those providers who have had appropriate training, and can demonstrate that they are able to perform them.

A set of core privileges for Gastroenterology might include the following:

- Privilege to Admit or Consult on Patients 18 Years or Older for Evaluation and Treatment of Diseases and Disorders of the Esophagus, Stomach, Small Intestine, and Colon, as well as the Liver, Biliary Tract, and Pancreas
- Privilege to Perform the following Procedures:
  - o Upper Gastrointestinal Endoscopy with Biopsy and Polypectomy, with Hemostasis of Bleeding Sources, including Bleeding Esophageal Varices
  - o Esophageal Dilatation by Balloon or Bougie
  - o Colonoscopy to the Cecum, including Biopsy, Polypectomy, and Hemostasis of Bleeding Sites
  - o Percutaneous Liver Biopsy
  - o Percutaneous Endoscopic Gastrostomy (PEG)
  - o Paracentesis
- Administration of Sedation, in Accordance with Hospital Policy

In addition, certain special privileges may be granted to those Gastroenterologists who demonstrate sufficient training and experience. These may include:

- Endoscopic Retrograde Cholangiopancreatography (ERCP), Diagnostic and Therapeutic
- Capsule Endoscopy
- Esophageal Manometry, Performance and Interpretation

If we now build a provider profile for a Gastroenterologist who has the core privileges, the profile in summary might look something like Table 3.1, below. Here we start with the Generic Profile detailed in Chapter 2, and add the core privileges, in italics.

Table 3.1 Gastroenterologist Profile draft

CATEGORY	MEASURE SUMMARY	ACGME CATEGORY
Volume	Volume of Discharges as Attending, Procedure Provider, Consultant	Patient Care
Acuity	Average CMI by MS-DRG and APR-DRG, as Attending and Procedure Provider	Patient Care
Clinical Outcome	Clinical Outcomes of Care, including Mortality, Complications, and Other Events, Risk Adjusted when Possible	Patient Care
Efficiency	Length of Stay, Acuity Adjusted Cost, Readmission Rates	Systems-Based Practice
Processes of Care	Core Measures, and Compliance with Other Best Practices; Drug and Blood Utilization	Patient Care
Privileges	*Upper GI Endoscopy* *Esophageal Dilatation* *Colonoscopy* *Percutaneous Liver Biopsy* *Percutaneous Endoscopic Gastrostomy* *Paracentesis*	*Patient Care; Systems-Based Practice*
Patient Satisfaction	Results of Patient Satisfaction Surveys; Validated Patient Complaints	Interpersonal and Communication Skills

continued >>

CATEGORY	MEASURE SUMMARY	ACGME CATEGORY
Citizenship	Timely Completion of Medical Records, including Discharge Summaries, Operative Notes, History/Physicals; Compliance with Medical Staff Bylaws, Rules, and Regulations; Internal Staff Surveys and Validated Complaints; Participation in Medical Staff Committees; Participation in In-House Officer Training Programs/Resident Education; CME Credits per Quarter	Professionalism, Medical Knowledge
Review	Count of All Cases Peer Reviewed, with Outcomes; Risk Management Claims Pending, and Settled or Pending; Review of Any Issues, including Invasive Procedure, Infection Control, Blood Usage, Pharmacy and Therapeutics, etc.	Practice-Based Learning and Improvement

An expanded view of the profile by privilege might look like Table 3.2.

Table 3.2 Gastroenterology Profile by Privilege

CATEGORY	MEASURE SUMMARY	ACGME CATEGORY
Privileges		
	Upper GI Endoscopy	
	Volume as Procedure Provider (Total)	Patient Care
	Emergent Cases, % Total	Patient Care
	Median Duration of Endoscopy in Minutes with Range	Systems-Based Practice
	No Findings (Normal), % Total	Patient Care
	Esophageal Dilatation	
	Volume as Procedure Provider (Total)	Patient Care
	Complications, Count and % Total	Patient Care
	Colonoscopy	
	Volume as Procedure Provider (Total)	Patient Care
	Emergent Cases, % Total	Patient Care
	Median Duration of Endoscopy in Minutes with Range	Systems-Based Practice
	Cases Examined to the Cecum, % Total	Patient Care
	No Findings (Normal), % Total	Patient Care
	Polypectomy, % Total	Patient Care
	Complications, Count and % Total	Patient Care

CATEGORY	MEASURE SUMMARY	ACGME CATEGORY
	Percutaneous Liver Biopsy	
	Volume as Procedure Provider (Total)	Patient Care
	Cases with Adequate Tissue for Diagnosis, Count and % Total	Patient Care
	Complications, Count and % Total	Patient Care
	Percutaneous Endoscopic Gastrostomy (PEG)	
	Volume as Procedure Provider (Total)	Patient Care
	Cases with Successful Tube Placement, Count and % Total	Patient Care
	Complications, Count and % Total	Patient Care
	Paracentesis	
	Volume as Procedure Provider (Total)	Patient Care
	Complications, Count and % Total	Patient Care

Note that with this focused approach, for each privilege, we include measures of Volume, Acuity, Outcome, Efficiency, and Processes of Care. Thus, the provider and her reviewer may view these measures clustered by each privilege, allowing better assessment of the provider's privilege-based performance. Remember that a central goal of the OPPE process is to determine whether to continue or amend the provider's privileges; setting up the profile on a privilege basis is aligned with this outcome.

The next consideration centers on how to start effectively and efficiently adding privilege-specific measures to the base Generic Profile, knowing that such changes cannot happen overnight. The following steps may provide a path for you:

- Assemble a team that includes Medical Staff leadership and appropriate Medical Staff Office members, including those who do credentialing/re-credentialing and Quality support. See Chapter 7.
- Review your current privileging policies and procedures. If you are using a core approach, you already have a good start. If your current approach needs to be revised, now is a good time to update these policies and procedures.

- Review the full scope of services offered by your facility, checking that the Medical Staff privileges match the services the hospital provides. Look for diagnoses and/or procedures that are high volume, high risk, or problem-prone ("Attributes," 2014). List these, and arrange them in descending order.

Follow the Pareto Principle, seeking a limited number of privileges that will cover the most patients. For example, consider the following hospital with an active Emergency Room with advanced Stroke and Heart Care, as well as standard Medical/Surgical Care, combined with a high volume Obstetrics service. If it has a specialty focus on Total Joint Replacement and Bariatric Surgery, an initial list might look like this:

- Treatment of Myocardial Infarction with Percutaneous Coronary Intervention [high volume, high risk]
- Acute Stroke Intervention [high risk, problem-prone]
- Delivery of Term Infants [high volume]
- Total Knee and Hip Replacement [high volume]
- Bariatric Surgery [high volume]

Start with Interventional Cardiology, looking at core privileges, and any high volume special privileges, in a manner similar to the example for Gastroenterology. Next, add procedures for the Acute Stroke Program, followed by Obstetrics (Vaginal Deliveries and C-Sections), and any special high risk procedures. Finally, add Orthopedic and Bariatric procedures. Basically, the process focuses on hospital services, starting with privileges that are high volume, high risk, and/or problem-prone.

Although the final goal is to have privilege-based metrics for all providers, if you start in this manner, you may be able to cover more than half of the patients and procedures in these top 5 areas.

Once you have prioritized privileges and specialties, determine the best metrics for each procedure based on input from your Medical Staff, national organizations, and published best practices.

Note that the data required for privilege-based measures may need to come from sources beyond those needed for the Generic Profile. For details on this, see Chapter 6. Most of the generic measures, with Medical and Surgical variants, are based on hospital discharge data from hospital administrative or quality systems. This administrative, or UB-04, data offers a great deal of insight into many provider performance areas. However, it may be difficult to get correct attribution or sufficient detail from administrative data to accurately track provider performance based on privileges. To expand your profiles beyond the Generic and into privileges, look to other data sources within your organization.

Begin this search by focusing on data that may be in stand-alone specialty data systems that support operative, endoscopy, or special procedures. For example, your Gastrointestinal Endoscopy Lab or the Cardiac Catheterization Suite may employ data systems built into their specialized equipment. Some systems include semi-automated report generation, combined with dictation capabilities, making data capture easier. Data on procedures and outcomes may already be entered into these systems, and can be a source for the measures on your provider profiles.

Next, look for any specialty databases used by your hospital. Many of the high volume/high risk procedure specialties belong to national organizations with specialty databases; in many cases, these specialties may already be collecting data and submitting it to a national database or organization. One of the earliest entries in this arena was by the Society of Thoracic Surgeons (STS), which collects detailed data on Cardiac Surgery. For more on specialty databases, see Chapter 6.

Once you have identified data sources, and matched them to the privilege groups, it is time to draft measures for each privilege, following the pattern – Volume, Acuity, Outcomes, Efficiency, and Processes of Care:

- **Volume:** This is probably the single most important metric for 2 reasons. First, high Volume has been shown to correlate with good performance (see Chapter 1). Second, Volume adds statistical Validity to metrics such as Mortality, Complications, and Patient Satisfaction. Put another way, a high Volume provider with high Mortality and Complication Rates will have a larger number of Complications, making his/her performance more evident. For a provider with 10 procedures a year, a 10% Complication Rate is just 1 Complication per year, which might slide through Peer Review. The same provider with 100 procedures per year and a 10% Complication Rate would have 10 Complications, almost 1 per month, enough to create a log jam in the Peer Review system, getting the attention of the Medical Staff.

- **Acuity:** This is a metric that looks for the "difficult cases" or situations that require greater skill. In the Upper GI Endoscopy measures, Emergent Cases as a Percentage of the Total is offered as a measure of Acuity or difficulty, on the assumption that emergency cases represent sicker patients often cared for under time pressure during off hours in acute care settings. However, the complexity of determining how 'sick' a patient is, and what this means for his or her provider, is inherently challenging (Yurkiewicz, 2014). Discovering how your hospital accounts for Acuity is vital; however, you may find that Mortality Rates, especially by service and given chronic conditions, may be used in determining patient Acuity ("Mortality rates," 2015).

- **Outcomes:** These measures may include Complication Rates, Delays in Discharge, and Returns (to Operating Room or other location) within 24-48 Hours Post Procedure. Ask leaders in each specialty to identify the red flags that tell them, "Something did not go right" with the procedure; see if these can be translated into measures. The Agency for Healthcare Research and Quality notes how central Care Outcomes are in Quality of Care assessments ("Selecting health outcome," 2014).

- **Efficiency:** By privilege, look for measures that reflect if things went smoothly and efficiently. Example metrics may include Time in the OR or Endoscopy Suite, or Costs Associated with a Procedure. Again, look to the Medical Staff for best practices and the key indicators of a smooth and efficient practice. Note that Efficiency and Quality correlate - unexpected events or problems consume time and resources. Likewise, the pursuit of providing high Quality Care often results in more increased Efficiency (Edwards, Silow-Carroll, & Lashbrook, 2011).

- **Processes of Care:** It can be a challenge to identify Process of Care metrics by privilege or procedure. Certainly for treatment of Myocardial Infarction, there are established processes, such as Aspirin at Admission, that are agreed upon and measured routinely. However, other Process measures may not be as supported by evidenced-based clinical care guidelines ("Selecting process measures," 2014). Still, for each privilege or process, it's important to look for "best steps" in its performance, including the elements that are necessary or that contribute to a good Outcomes. For example, consider including Informed Consent Obtained Prior to a Procedure, Providing Discharge Instructions, or Using a Standard Checklist Prior to or During a Procedure. Any step that decreases Risk and contributes to Safety can be considered a Process of Care element for these metrics.

Examples Based on Common High Volume Specialties

Now that we have walked through some possible privilege-based metrics for Gastroenterology, let's look at some of the more common specialties, roughly in descending order of Volume within an average community hospital. For each specialty, we have researched how core privileges may be defined, and suggested metrics that might reflect performance of these privileges. The following is offered as a guideline or a place to start, with the understanding that the profiling process is by and for the Medical Staff, who must both approve the measures and provide assurance that they match the hospital's scope of practice, consistent with the needs of the community it serves.

Orthopedics: Orthopedics is a common and important specialty devoted to the diagnosis and treatment of diseases and injuries of the skeletal system, its joints, and associated structures. At many hospitals, it is the highest Volume surgical specialty based on number of procedures performed ("High volume hospitals," 2011). It will likely be high on your list of specialties when you create privilege-based metrics.

As with other specialties, it's important to realize that the core privileges tend to match what an Orthopedic Surgeon is trained to do during her residency, including treating fractures and replacing joints. In addition to the core privileges, there are specialty categories, which vary by the hospital's scope of practice. For Orthopedics, common subspecialties include Hand and Spine. In addition, there are special categories of procedures that require separate training and/or certification. Administration of Procedural Sedation and Fluoroscopy are commonly included in this list.

The list of procedures for the core privilege categories can be extensive. When you review a large list, look for 2 distinct features: the high volume procedures at your hospital that match the core; and lower volume procedures that are high risk or problem-prone, and warrant monitoring for volume and outcome. In Orthopedics, Proximal Amputation for Cancer might fall into this latter category. Chances are, the high volume procedures will include Total Knee and Hip Replacement, probably followed by Repair of Hip Fracture, and Treatment of the Results of Trauma, including Setting Long Bones. Tracking a few high volume procedures may be both an efficient and valid monitoring strategy, since these procedures may require the same basic skills as the host of individual procedures on the core list.

See Table 3.3, Orthopedics, for a sample list of Orthopedics privileges, and associated metrics.

Obstetrics/Gynecology: One of the highest Volume specialties in many hospitals is Obstetrics. This is due in part to the fact that the delivery of an infant is safest in a unit associated with advanced Obstetrical and Neonatal Services, which in turn require a high volume center. Most Obstetricians also practice Gynecology, but as these providers age, they may restrict their practice to Gynecology only, given the physical demands of delivering infants 24 hours per day, 7 days per week. Some Gynecologists may specialize in Gynecologic Oncology or Fertility. If one of the subspecialty services is high Volume, such as Fertility, it may warrant creation of a separate profile for that subspecialty. Again, look at the services that your hospital provides, using this information to determine how many unique profiles you will need, and what metrics to build. See Table 3.4, OB/GYN, for privileges and metrics associated with Obstetrics/Gynecology.

Pediatrics and Neonatology: If your hospital offers Obstetrics to a high Volume of patients, then you also likely provide a Neonatology Service, with the Volume of newborn infants in line with the number of deliveries. You may or may not offer a Pediatric Service, depending on your community; larger communities may have a fully dedicated Pediatric Hospital. See Table 3.5, Pediatrics and Neonatology, for an example of how to structure metrics for these specialties.

General Surgery: General Surgery is probably next in line for privilege-based metrics. In broad strokes, Surgeons either admit electively to perform

Surgery, or provide Surgical Services for the acutely ill or injured who are admitted emergently. In either case, the predominant activity of a Surgeon is Surgery, for which he is granted specific privileges. Monitoring performance by privilege will provide a fairly accurate picture of a Surgeon's Volume and Outcomes.

One of the challenges of General Surgery as a category is that General Surgeons tend to sub-specialize both during training and during the course of practice. Forty years ago, a General Surgeon's activity included all Surgery in the abdomen, plus Breast Surgery. Although this continues in some facilities today, General Surgeons may specialize in only Breast, Bariatrics, Pancreatic and Liver, Transplantation, or Colon and Rectal Surgery. Depending on the scope of practice at your hospital, you may be able to cover all privileges in a single profile, or may choose to create separate profiles to match the Surgeon's activity. For example, you may decide to create a profile just for Bariatics, or just for Colon and Rectal Surgery.

Note that for General Surgery, the special privilege categories include newer robotic approaches to traditional surgery where special training and experience with specific equipment is required. Again, the inclusion of any special privilege in a profile depends on the scope of services at your hospital. Remember that the Medical Staff can only be granted privileges for procedures which can be done at your hospital. If you do not have robotic systems in your Operating Rooms, then no one should have privileges to Perform Robotic Surgery, even if specific providers have proper training and experience in this area.

Table 3.6, General Surgery, provides an example of privilege-based metrics for General Surgeons in a moderate sized community hospital with limited demand for sub-specialties. Note that we also have created profiles for the following 2 subspecialties: Bariatrics and Transplantation. For additional surgical subspecalities, such as Urology, Head and Neck Surgery, Vascular Surgery, and Cardiac Surgery, start with the General Surgery template, and customize it to meet your specific needs.

Hospital Medicine: Over the past 15 years, a progressive shift in inpatient medical care has occurred. The transition from an older model, where Internists and General Practitioners cared for both inpatient and outpatients, shuttling back and forth from their offices to the hospital, to a newer model in which Primary Care Physicians stay in the office, and inpatient care of their patient population is performed by a cadre of providers who specialize only in inpatient care, has occurred. It is likely that your hospital has Hospitalist groups; in turn, each Hospitalist group may have variable contractual obligations for services provided. Some research indicates that hospitals that contract Hospitalist groups often experience increased Efficiency (Edwards, Silow-Carroll, & Lashbrook, 2011).

Again, the Hospitalist profiles should reflect the metrics on the Generic Profile outlined in Chapter 2, plus metrics based on specific privileges not covered in the Generic Profile. The privileges granted to Hospitalists vary by hospital, depending on the scope of services provided by these providers. See Table 3.7, Hospital Medicine/Internal Medicine. Note that these privileges and associated metrics can also serve for independent Internists, including those who are not part of a Hospitalist group, depending on the structure of your Medical Staff.

Cardiology: Today, inpatient Cardiology tends to be high Volume and interventional. The current standard of practice for treating ST Elevation Acute Myocardial Infarction (STEMI) is Thrombolytics within 30 Minutes of Arrival (door to drug time), or Angioplasty/Stent Placement within 90 Minutes (door to balloon time). Coronary Arteriography with Intervention has dominated the treatment landscape recently, requiring Cardiac Catheterization laboratories and Interventional Cardiologists to be available 24 hours a day, 7 days a week. When looking for privilege-based measures, start with the Interventional Cardiologists, due to the sheer Volume of patients they may serve, looking for their privileges in the Cardiac Cath Lab. See Table 3.8, Cardiology, for an example of a mid- to large hospital with an active Emergency Room.

Critical Care/Pulmonology: Critical Care Medicine includes specialists who treat patients in the ICU and CCU, covering all aspects of acute and emergency care for the critically injured and ill ("The intensive care,"2014). As a branch of Medicine, it is concerned with the diagnosis and management of life-threatening conditions that require care by sophisticated, skilled providers who have been trained to identify and respond to needs in the most stressful of situations. Pulmonology aligns well with the Critical Care service arena, as it focuses on the chest and the management of patients who need life support and mechanical ventilation. It is logical to combine these 2 specialties in many situations. Note that the other specialty commonly involved with Critical Care is Anesthesiology; see Chapter 4. See Table 3.9 for an example of metrics for Critical Care/Pulmonology based on core privileges.

Behavioral Health/Psychiatry: Behavioral Health has become, in many areas, the more accepted or standard term associated with the practice of Psychiatry and Psychology. Behavioral Health includes the treatment and prevention of mental illness, as well as substance abuse and addictions. The privilege list will vary depending on the services provided by your facility, and if patients are treated as inpatient, outpatient, or both. In addition, provision of services to court-ordered patients or those who have been mandated to receive psychiatric evaluations and/or care may require special privileges. Further variation may exist in terms of substance abuse treatment methodologies, and complications/comorbidities of the patient population.

The ability to assess patients via a psycho-social evaluation and to take the patient's case history is typically the starting point of this field's scope of care. The diagnosis of mental disorders is governed by the criteria detailed in diagnostic manuals; the most accepted of these is the Diagnostic and Statistical Manual of Mental Disorders (DSM), fifth edition (DSM-5), which was published in 2013 ("About DSM-5," 2014). See Table 3.10, Behavioral Health/Psychiatry, for a sample starting point for this specialty.

Rehabilitation/Physical Medicine: Physical Medicine and Rehabilitation, often shortened to PM&R, also known as Physiatry, is a branch of Medicine with a goal of enhancing/restoring functional ability and quality of life to those with physical impairments and/or disabilities. Some specialists in this field focus on restoring function to people with injuries to the muscles, bones, tissues, and nervous system. Others may work primarily with patients who have spinal cord injuries, amputations, sports injuries, or traumatic brain injuries. Common subspecialties include Hospice and Palliative Care, Neuromuscular Medicine, Pain Medicine, and Sports Medicine. Given the scope of services delivered by those who practice PM&R, it is clear that at times they will work closely with providers in other fields including Neurology and Surgery. See Table 3.11.

Summary

In this chapter, we have begun the process of adding privilege-based metrics to the Generic Profile. We have explored our priorities associated with privilege-based evaluation, and we offered an array of metrics associated with high volume specialties that may be relevant to your hospital.

Next Steps

Next, we will address 4 of the more challenging specialties for profiling: Pathology, Radiology, Emergency Medicine, and Anesthesiology. These are high volume and essential for an active multispecialty hospital, but lack a simple standardized approach to gathering performance data by specialty. In Chapter 4, we will examine each of these specialties, along with recommendations for data sources and metrics to meet their profiling needs.

Reference List:

"About DSM-V." (2014). American Psychiatric Association. Retrieved from http://www.dsm5.org/about/pages/default.aspx

"Attributes of core performance measures and associated evaluation criteria." (2014). The Joint Commission. Retrieved from http://www.jointcommission.org/assets/1/18/Attributes_of_Core_Performance_Measures_and_Associated_Evaluation_Criteria.pdf

"Clinical privilege white paper: Addiction medicine." (2012). HCPro, *Credentialing Resource Center Journal.* Retrieved from http://www.hcpro.com/content/278280.pdf

Colwell, J. (2010). The rise of the hospitalist. *American College of Physicians: Hospitalist.* Retrieved from http://www.acphospitalist.org/archives/2010/06/neuro.htm

"Core/bundled privileges." (2008). The Joint Commission: Medical Staff CAMH/Hospitals, Standards FAQ Details. Retrieved from http://www.jointcommission.org/mobile/standards_information/jcfaqdetails.aspx?StandardsFAQId=42&StandardsFAQChapterId=74

"Credentialing and privileging." (2014). HCPro. Retrieved from http://www.hcpro.com/credentialing-Privileging

"Delineation of privileges." (2012). University of Michigan Hospitals and Health Centers. Retrieved from http://www.med.umich.edu/mss/pdf/OBGYN%20New.pdf

"Delineation of privileges, department of pediatrics, division of pediatric hospitalist—pediatric hospitalist." (2014). University of Michigan Hospitals and Health Centers. Retrieved from http://www.med.umich.edu/mss/pdf/ped-hospitalist.pdf

"Delineation of privileges for child psychiatry, department of psychiatry." (2014). Yale-New Haven Hospital. Retrieved from http://www.ynhh.org/vSiteManager/Upload/Docs/Med_Staff_Applicants/BH/Del/Delineation_of_Privileges_for_Child_Psychiatry_2014.pdf

"Detroit Medical Center, department of family medicine, delineation of privileges." (2009). Detroit Medical Center. Retrieved from https://www.dmc.org/upload/docs/MA_Privileges_Membership/Family%20Medicine%20DOP%20DMC.pdf

Edwards, J.N., Silow-Carroll, S., & Lashbrook, A. (2011). Achieving efficiency: Lessons from four top-performing hospitals. The Commonwealth Fund. Retrieved from http://www.commonwealthfund.org/~/media/Files/Publications/Case%20Study/2011/Jul/1528_Edwards_achieving_efficiency_synthesis_four_top_hosps_v3.pdf

"Fort Hamilton Hospital, specialty: Cardiology-Department of Medicine, delineation of privileges." (2013). Fort Hamilton Hospital, Kettering Health. Retrieved from http://www.ketteringhealth.org/medstaff/pdffhh/physicianprivileges/Cardiology.pdf

"Guidelines for institutions granting privileges." (2014). SAGES: Society for American Gastrointestinal and Endoscopic Surgeons. Retrieved from http://www.sages.org/

"High volume hospitals improve orthopedic outcomes." (2011). Hospital for Special Surgery. Retrieved from http://www.hss.edu/newsroom_high-volume-hospitals-improve-Orthopedic-outcomes.asp

"Hospital-based psychiatric services." (2014). UC San Diego Health System. Retrieved from https://health.ucsd.edu/specialties/psych/Pages/adult-inpatient.aspx

"Hospital privileging for family physicians." (2015). American Academy of Family Physicians. Retrieved from http://www.aafp.org/practice-management/administration/privileging.html

"Huntington Hospital delineation of privileges, comprehensive pain management privileges." (2014). Huntington Hospital. Retrieved from http://www.huntingtonhospital.com/Resource.ashx?sn=ComprehensivePainManagementPrivileges

"Kaleida Health: Delineation of privileges-pediatrics and pediatric subspecialties." (2011). Kaleida Health. Retrieved from http://www.kaleidahealth.org/providers/support/DOP/PED-050111.pdf

"Midland Memorial Hospital: Delineation of privileges, interventional cardiology." (2012). Midland Memorial Hospital. Retrieved from http://www.midland-memorial.com/Resources/15365/FileRepository/For%20Physicians/Privileges/Delineation_of_Privileges_Interventional_Cardiology.pdf

"Mortality rates by service." (2015). Rush University Medical Center. Retrieved from https://www.rush.edu/quality-care/quality-rush/quality-and-safety-rush/mortality-rates-service-quality-care-rush

"Physical medicine and rehabilitation clinical privileges." (2013). University Hospital and Health System, University of Mississippi Medical Center. Retrieved from http://www.umc.edu/uploadedFiles/UMCedu/Content/Administration/Business_Services/Medical_Staff_Services/New_Faculty/ORT%20-%20Physical%20Medicine%20and%20Rehabilitation%20Clinical%20Privileges_rev04032013.pdf

"Selecting health outcome measures for clinical quality measurement." (2014). Agency for Healthcare Research and Quality. Retrieved from http://www.qualitymeasures.ahrq.gov/tutorial/HealthOutcomeMeasure.aspx

"Selecting process measures for clinical quality measurement." (2014). Agency for Healthcare Research and Quality. Retrieved from http://www.qualitymeasures. ahrq.gov/tutorial/ProcessMeasure.aspx

"The intensive care professionals." (2014). The Society of Critical Care Medicine. Retrieved from http://www.sccm.org/Pages/default.aspx

"Yale-New Haven Hospital core privileges, pulmonology/critical care medicine." (2014). Yale-New Haven Hospital. Retrieved from http://www.ynhh.org/vSiteManager/Upload/Images/Professionals/Pulmonology.pdf

Yale, S.H., Hansotia, P., Knapp, D., & Ehrfurth, J. (2003). Neurologic conditions: Assessing medical fitness to drive. *Clinical Medicine and Research*. Retrieved from http://www.ncbi.nlm.nih.gov/pmc/articles/PMC1069044/

Yurkiewicz, I. (2014). Sick or not sick? Handing the reality of inpatient medicine. KevinMD.com. Retrieved from http://www.kevinmd.com/ blog/2014/11/sick-sick-handling-reality-inpatient-medicine.html

Table 3.3 Orthopedics

Core	**Definition:** AEDTC[1] All Ages CII[2] of the Extremities, Spine, and Associated Structures, with Medical, Surgical, or Physical Means. **Procedures include:** Amputation, Arthroscopy, Biopsy, Bone Grafts, Carpal Tunnel Decompression, Closed/Open Reduction of Fractures, Dislocations, with Fixation. Excision, Debridement, Reconstruction. Arthroplasty of Knee, Hip, or Shoulder. Muscle and Tendon Repair.	
	Privilege Core	Metrics
	Total Knee Replacement	Volume, Clinical Outcomes, Efficiency, Processes of Care, Reviews
	Total Hip Replacement	Volume, Clinical Outcomes, Efficiency, Processes of Care, Reviews
Hand	**Definition:** AEDTC All Ages CII of the Structures of the Upper Extremity Directly Affecting the Form and Function of the Hand and Wrist with Medical, Surgical, and Physical Means. **Procedures include:** Arthroplasty of Large or Small Joints, Wrists, or Hand, including Implants, Bone Grafting, Carpal Tunnel Decompression, Fracture Fixation with Compression Plates or Wires, Open and Closed Reductions of Fractures, Tendon Release, Repair, Fixation or Reconstruction. Repair of Rheumatoid Arthritis Deformity, Skin Grafts, Repair of Lacerations, and Treatment of Infections.	
	Privilege Hand	Metrics
	Hand and Wrist Procedures	Volume, Clinical Outcomes, Efficiency, Processes of Care, Reviews
Spine	**Definition:** AEDTC All Ages CII Spinal Column Disease, Disorders and Injuries by Medical, Physical, and Surgical Methods. **Procedures include:** Laminectomies, Fixation and Reconstructive Procedures of the Spine and Its Contents. Endoscopic Minimally Invasive Spinal Surgery. Management of Traumatic, Congenital, Developmental, Infectious, Metabolic, Degenerative, and Rheumatologic Disorders of the Spine. Spinal Cord Surgery for Decompression of the Spinal Cord or Spinal Canal, Rhizotomy, Cordotomy, Dorsal Root Entry Zone Lesions, Tethered Spinal Cord or Other Congenital Anomalies.	
	Privilege Spine	Metrics
	Dorsal and Lumbar Fusion	Volume, Clinical Outcomes, Efficiency, Processes of Care, Reviews
	Intervertebral Disc Excision and Decompression	Volume, Clinical Outcomes, Efficiency, Processes of Care, Reviews
Special	Percutaneous Lumbar Discectomy	Volume, Clinical Outcomes, Efficiency, Processes of Care, Reviews
	Balloon Kyphoplasty	Volume, Clinical Outcomes, Efficiency, Processes of Care, Reviews
	Artificial Disc Replacement	Volume, Clinical Outcomes, Efficiency, Processes of Care, Reviews
	Administration of Sedation and Analgesia	Volume, Clinical Outcomes, Efficiency, Processes of Care, Reviews
	Flouroscopy	Volume, Clinical Outcomes, Efficiency, Processes of Care, Reviews

[1] Admit, Evaluate, Diagnose, Treat and Provide Consultation
[2] Conditions, Illnesses and Injuries

Table 3.4 Obstetrics and Gynecology

Core	**Definition:** AEDTC Adolescent and Adult Women to Provide Medical and Surgical Care of the Reproductive System to include Pregnancy and Medical Disorders Complicating Pregnancy. **Procedures include:** Management of Normal and High Risk Pregnancies to Include Vaginal or Cesarean Delivery. Procedures Associated with Pregnancy and Delivery, including Amniocentesis; Application and Interpretation of Fetal Monitoring; Breech Delivery, Manual Removal of Placenta and Uterine Curettage; Obstetrical Ultrasound; Induction and Augmentation of Labor.	
	Privilege Obstetrics	Metrics
	Vaginal Delivery	Volume, Clinical Outcomes, Efficiency, Processes of Care, Reviews
	Cesarean Delivery	Volume, Clinical Outcomes, Efficiency, Processes of Care, Reviews
	Induction of Labor	Volume, Clinical Outcomes (% Vaginal Delivery, % C-Section), Efficiency, Processes of Care, Reviews
	Amniocentesis/Fetal Maturity Study	Volume, Clinical Outcomes, Efficiency, Processes of Care, Reviews
	Post-Partum Tubal Sterilization	Volume, Clinical Outcomes, Efficiency, Processes of Care, Reviews
Gynecology	**Definition**: AEDTC Women of All Ages with Disorders of the Reproductive and Genitourinary System **Procedures include:** Uterine and Adnexal Procedures, Uterine and Adnexal Procedures for Ovarian and Adnexal Malignancy, Pelvic Evisceration/Radical Hysterectomy	
	Privilege Gynecology	Metrics
	Uterine and Adnexal Procedures, [% with Hysterectomy, % Hysterectomy for Benign Disease]	Volume, Clinical Outcomes, Efficiency, Processes of Care (% Open, % Laparoscopic), Reviews
	Uterine and Adnexal Procedures for Ovarian and Adnexal Malignancy	Volume, Clinical Outcomes, Efficiency, Processes of Care, Reviews
	Pelvic Evisceration/Radical Hysterectomy	Volume, Clinical Outcomes, Efficiency, Processes of Care, Reviews
Special	Pelvic Prolapse Repair with Mesh	Volume, Clinical Outcomes, Efficiency, Processes of Care, Reviews
	Advanced Fertility Therapy	Volume, Clinical Outcomes, Efficiency, Processes of Care, Reviews
	High Complexity Operative Vaginal Delivery	Volume, Clinical Outcomes, Efficiency, Processes of Care, Reviews

References: "Delineation of privileges," (2012).

Table 3.5 Pediatrics/Neonatal

Core	**Definition**: AEDTC Patients from Birth to 21 Years with Acute and Chronic Disease, Including Major Complicated Illnesses and Routine Newborn Care. **Procedures include:** Attendance at Delivery to Assume Care of Normal Newborns, Frenulectomy, Incision and Drainage of Abscess, Burns: Superficial and Partial Thickness, Arthrocentesis and Joint Injection, Management of Uncomplicated Minor Closed Fractures and Dislocations, Peripheral Nerve Blocks, Skin Biopsy, Lumbar Puncture, Suture Uncomplicated Laceration. Venipuncture, Arterial Puncture, Bladder Catheterization, Lumbar Puncture; Laceration Repairs; Care of Infants, (including Pre-term Infants) in Nursery; Consultation of PICU Patients; Myringotomy, Tympanocentesis, Delivery Room Management and Resuscitation; Arterial Puncture, and Interpretation of Blood Gas Results.	
	Privilege Core	Metrics
	Attendance at Delivery	Volume, Clinical Outcomes, Efficiency, Processes of Care, Reviews
	Lumbar Puncture	Volume, Clinical Outcomes, Efficiency, Processes of Care, Reviews
	Care of Full Term Newborns, Late Pre-Term Newborns in Level I Nursery	Volume, Clinical Outcomes, Efficiency, Processes of Care, Reviews
	Venipuncture	Volume, Clinical Outcomes, Efficiency, Processes of Care, Reviews
Special	Adolescent Medicine	Volume, Clinical Outcomes, Efficiency, Processes of Care, Reviews
	Pediatric Allergy/Immunology	Volume, Clinical Outcomes, Efficiency, Processes of Care, Reviews
	Newborn/Pediatric Endocrinology	Volume, Clinical Outcomes, Efficiency, Processes of Care, Reviews
	Pediatric Hematology/Oncology	Volume, Clinical Outcomes, Efficiency, Processes of Care, Reviews

Neonatal/Perinatal		
Core	**Definition**: AEDTC Newborns with Severe and Complex Life-Threatening Problems such as Respiratory Failure, Shock, Congenital Abnormalities, and Sepsis. Provide Consultation to Mothers with High-Risk Pregnancies, <32 Weeks. **Procedures include:** Attendance at Delivery of High Risk Newborns. Cardiac Life Support, Endotracheal Intubation, Exchange Transfusion, Insertion and Management of Central Lines and Chest Tubes, Lumbar Puncture, Paracentesis, Thoracentesis, Pericardiocentesis, Peripheral Arterial Catheterization, Peritoneal Dialysis, Umbilical Catheterization, Ventilator Care of Infants.	
	Privilege Core	Metrics
	NICU Volume and Outcomes as Attending	Volume, Clinical Outcomes, Efficiency, Processes of Care, Reviews
	Endotracheal Intubation	Volume, Clinical Outcomes, Efficiency, Processes of Care, Reviews
	Exchange Transfusion	Volume, Clinical Outcomes, Efficiency, Processes of Care, Reviews
	Central Line Insertion	Volume, Clinical Outcomes, Efficiency, Processes of Care, Reviews
	Chest Tube Insertion	Volume, Clinical Outcomes, Efficiency, Processes of Care, Reviews
	Peritoneal Dialysis	Volume, Clinical Outcomes, Efficiency, Processes of Care, Reviews
	Ventilator Management, Days	Volume, Clinical Outcomes, Efficiency, Processes of Care, Reviews

References: "Kaleida Health," (2011).

Table 3.6 General Surgery

Core	**Definition**: AEDTC Patients of All Ages for Diseases, Disorders, and Injuries of the Alimentary Tract, the Abdomen and Its Contents, Extremities, Breast, Skin, and Soft Tissue, Head and Neck, and Endocrine Systems. **Procedures include:** Procedures (Open or via Laparoscopy) on the Abdominal Contents, including Appendectomy, Bowel Resection to Include Gastrectomy and Colectomy, Drainage of Abscesses, and Splenectomy. Surgery on the Breast, including Mastectomy. Pancreatic Resection. Transabdominal Esophagectomy, Hepatic Resection. Surgery on Thyroid and Parathyroid. Vein Ligation and Stripping	
	Privilege Core	Metrics
	Total Laparotomies	Volume, Clinical Outcomes (% Open, % Laparoscopic), Efficiency, Processes of Care, Reviews
	Pancreatic Resection	Volume, Clinical Outcomes, Efficiency, Processes of Care, Reviews
	Colectomy	Volume, Clinical Outcomes, Efficiency, Processes of Care, Reviews
	Thyroid/Parathyroid Surgery	Volume, Clinical Outcomes, Efficiency, Processes of Care, Reviews
	Vein Ligation and Stripping	Volume, Clinical Outcomes, Efficiency, Processes of Care, Reviews
	Cholecystectomy	Volume, Clinical Outcomes, Efficiency, Processes of Care, Reviews
	Splenectomy	Volume, Clinical Outcomes, Efficiency, Processes of Care, Reviews
Bariatrics	**Definition:** AEDTC for Patients of All Ages for Surgical Treatment of Obesity. **Procedures include:** Open or Laparoscopic Performance of Surgery on the Stomach and Intestine to Reduce Weight by Limiting Intake or Absorption of Nutrients, including Procedures Requiring Transection of the GI Tract (Laparoscopic Roux-en-Y Gastric Bypass, Sleeve Gastrectomy, etc.) or Gastric Banding.	
	Privilege Bariatrics	Metrics
	Procedures Requiring Transection of the GI Tract	Volume, Clinical Outcomes, Efficiency, Processes of Care, Reviews
	Gastric Banding	Volume, Clinical Outcomes, Efficiency, Processes of Care, Reviews
Transplantation	**Definition**: Multi-Organ Abdominal; Kidney; Liver; Pancreas Transplantation, Preparation, and Post-Surgery Care. **Procedures include:** Liver Transplant, Kidney-Pancreas Transplant, Pancreas Alone Transplant (PAT), Living Donor Kidney, Deceased Donor Kidney, Islet Cell Pancreatic Surgery/Whipple Procedure with Islet Cell Transplantation	
	Privilege Transplantation	Metrics
	Liver Transplant	Volume, Clinical Outcomes, Efficiency, Processes of Care, Reviews
	Kidney-Pancreas	Volume, Clinical Outcomes, Efficiency, Processes of Care, Reviews
Special	Robotic Surgery: Surgery per the Core Definitions, Performed by Robotic Techniques	Volume, Clinical Outcomes, Efficiency, Processes of Care, Reviews
	Endoscopy	Volume, Clinical Outcomes, Efficiency, Processes of Care, Reviews
	Procedural Sedation	Volume, Clinical Outcomes, Efficiency, Processes of Care, Reviews

References: "Guidelines," 2014.

Table 3.7 Hospital Medicine/Internal Medicine, Pediatric Hospitalist and Neurohospitalist

Core	**Definition:** AEDTC of Patients Ages Birth though 16 Years and Older for Nonsurgical Treatment Of General Medical Problems, including (Pre- and Post-Operative Care as Needed. **Procedures include:** Lumbar Puncture, Joint Aspiration/Injection, Incision and Drainage of Abscess, Diagnostic Proctoscopy, Thoracentesis, Abdominal Paracentesis; Drawing of Arterial Blood Gases, Management of Burns, Superficial and Partial Thickness; Excision of Skin and Subcutaneous Tumors, Nodules, and Lesions; Insertion and Management of Central Venous Catheters and Arterial Lines; Local Anesthetic Techniques; Nasogastric Intubation, Endotracheal Intubation and Advanced Life Support; Placement of Peripheral Venous Line, Interpretation of EKGs.	
	Privilege Core	Metrics
	Insertion of Central Venous Catheters	Volume, Clinical Outcomes, Efficiency, Processes of Care, Reviews
	Abdominal Paracentesis	Volume, Clinical Outcomes, Efficiency, Processes of Care, Reviews
	Nasogastric Intubation	Volume, Clinical Outcomes, Efficiency, Processes of Care, Reviews
Pediatric Hospitalist	**Definition:** EDTC of Patients Birth to Young Adult in the Inpatient Hospital Setting. **Procedures include:** Endotracheal Intubation; Simple Removal of Foreign Bodies from Ears/Nose; Gastric Lavage; Immunizations; Subcutaneous, Intradermal, Intramuscular, and Joint Aspiration Injections; Peripheral Arterial Puncture; Venous Aspirations; Place Central Lines; Monitor Vital Signs	
	Privilege Pediatric Hospitalist	Metrics
	Endotracheal Intubation	Volume, Clinical Outcomes, Efficiency, Processes of Care, Reviews
	Removal of Foreign Body from Ears/Nose	Volume, Clinical Outcomes, Efficiency, Processes of Care, Reviews
	Gastric Lavage	Volume, Clinical Outcomes, Efficiency, Processes of Care, Reviews
	Immunizations	Volume, Clinical Outcomes, Efficiency, Processes of Care, Reviews
	Subcutaneous, Intradermal, Intramuscular, and Joint Aspiration Injections	Volume, Clinical Outcomes, Efficiency, Processes of Care, Reviews
	Peripheral Arterial Puncture	Volume, Clinical Outcomes, Efficiency, Processes of Care, Reviews
	Venous Aspirations	Volume, Clinical Outcomes, Efficiency, Processes of Care, Reviews
	Place Central Lines	Volume, Clinical Outcomes, Efficiency, Processes of Care, Reviews
	Monitor Vital Signs	Volume, Clinical Outcomes, Efficiency, Processes of Care, Reviews

Neurohospitalist	**Definition**: EDTC of Patients Needing Neurological Care/Services in the ICU and in Other Hospital Environments; Order and Interpret Neurological Tests; Monitor Neurological Functioning **Procedures include:** Neurological Functional Testing; Neurological Monitoring; Implement and Monitor Neurological Treatment; Prepare Patients for Rehabilitative Treatments	
	Privilege Neurology	Metrics
	Neurological Function Testing	Volume, Clinical Outcomes, Efficiency, Processes of Care, Reviews
	Neurological Monitoring	Volume, Clinical Outcomes, Efficiency, Processes of Care, Reviews
	Implement and Monitor Neurological Treatment	Volume, Clinical Outcomes, Efficiency, Processes of Care, Reviews
	Prepare Patients for Rehabilitative Treatments	Volume, Clinical Outcomes, Efficiency, Processes of Care, Reviews
Special	EEG (Electromyography)	Volume, Clinical Outcomes, Efficiency, Processes of Care, Reviews
	Assess/Manage Persistent Vegetative State	Volume, Clinical Outcomes, Efficiency, Processes of Care, Reviews
	PET Studies	Volume, Clinical Outcomes, Efficiency, Processes of Care, Reviews
	Botulism Toxin Treatment	Volume, Clinical Outcomes, Efficiency, Processes of Care, Reviews

References: "Delineation of privileges-department of pediatrics," 2014.

Table 3.8 Cardiology

Core	**Definition:** AEDTC Patients Presenting with Diseases of the Heart, Lungs, and Blood Vessels and Manage Complex Cardiac Conditions. Assess, Stabilize, and Determine Disposition of Patients **Procedures include:** Adult Transthoracic Echocardiography; Ambulatory Electrocardiology Monitor Interpretation; Cardioversion (Electrical, Elective); Tilt Table Testing; Temporary Transvenous Pacemaker Insertion; Pericardiocentesis; Insertion and Management of Thromlolytic Agents and Antithrombolytic Agents, Placement and Management of Central Venous Lines, Pulmonary Artery Catheters, and Arterial Lines	
	Privilege Core	**Metrics**
	Adult Transthoracic Echocardiography	Volume, Clinical Outcomes, Efficiency, Processes of Care, Reviews
	Ambulatory Electrocardiology Monitor Interpretation	Volume, Clinical Outcomes, Efficiency, Processes of Care, Reviews
	Cardioversion (Electrical, Elective)	Volume, Outcome (Percentage of Success by Type of Rhyme, Processes: Compliance with Protocol, Review
	Tilt Table Testing	Volume, Clinical Outcomes, Efficiency, Processes of Care, Reviews
	Temporary Transvenous Pacemaker Insertion	Volume, Clinical Outcomes, Efficiency, Processes of Care, Reviews
	Periocardiocentesis	Volume, Clinical Outcomes, Efficiency, Processes of Care, Reviews
	Insertion and Management of Thrombolytic Agents and Antithrombotic Agents	Volume, Clinical Outcomes, Efficiency, Processes of Care, Reviews
	Placement and Management of Central Venous Lines, Pulmonary Artery Catheters, and Arterial Lines	Volume by Access Site, Outcome: Complications Including Infection Rate, Process: Compliance with Protocol, Review
Invasive Interventional Cardiology	**Definition:** Admit, Evaluate, Consult, and Treat Patients who Present with Acute or Chronic Heart Disease and Who May Require Invasive Diagnostic Procedures and Intervention as Necessary. **Procedures include:** Use of Intracoronary Doppler and Flow Wire; Percutaneous Coronary Intervention; Placement of Intracoronary Stents; Intravascular Ultrasound of Coronaries; Percutaneous Coronary Atherectomy; Coronary Angiography	
	Privilege Int Cardiology	**Metrics**
	Coronary Angiography: Diagnostic Only	Volume; Outcome: % Normal Study, Complications including Bleeding and Hematoma; Processes: Compliance with Protocols; Review
	Coronary Angiography: Interventional to Open Occluded Arteries	Volume by Indication and Type of Procedure, Outcome: % Open Artery, Complications Including Bleeding and Discharge to OR for CABG or Vascular Repair, Process: Compliance with Protocol, Review
	Myocardial Biopsy	Volume by Indication, Outcome: % Normal, Process: Compliance with Protocol of Care, Review

Electrophysiology	**Definition**: Admit, Evaluate, Diagnose, Treat, and Provide Consultation to Patients 16 Years and Older with Heart Rhythm Disorders. **Procedures include:** Perform Invasive Diagnostic and Therapeutic Cardiac Electrophysiology Procedures.	
	Privilege Electrophysiology	Metrics
	Insertion and Management of Pacemakers and Automatic Implantable Cardioverter Defibrillators	Volume by Type of Device and Indication, Outcome: Complications including Infection, Process: Compliance with Protocol, Review
	Interpretation of Electrophysiology Studies	Volume by Type of Study, Results of Double-Readings, Process: Turnaround Time; Review
	Therapeutic Catheter Ablation	Volume, Outcome: % Successful, Complications. Process: Compliance with Protocols, Time of Procedures (Mean, Median, Outliers, and/or Distribution, Review
Special	Fluoroscopy	Volume, Clinical Outcomes, Efficiency, Processes of Care, Reviews
	Procedural Sedation	Volume, Clinical Outcomes, Efficiency, Processes of Care, Reviews
	Cardiac CT Angiogram	Volume, Clinical Outcomes, Efficiency, Processes of Care, Reviews
	Transesophageal Echocardiography (TEE)	Volume, Clinical Outcomes, Efficiency, Processes of Care, Reviews

References: "Fort Hamilton," 2013; "Midland Memorial," 2012

Table 3.9 Critical Care/Pulmonary

Core	**Definition:** Admit, Evaluate, Diagnose, Treat, and Provide Consultation to Critically Ill Patients and Patients Presenting with Conditions, Disorders, and Diseases of the Organs of the Thorax or Chest; the Lungs and Airways; Cardiovascular and Tracheobronchial Systems; Esophagus and Other Mediastinal Contents, Diaphragm, and Circulatory System. **Procedures include:** Diagnostic Abdominal Paracentesis; Diagnostic Lumbar Puncture; Peripheral Arterial Puncture; Diagnostic Thoracentesis; Fiberoptic Bronchospcopy; Endotracheal Intubation, including Airway Maintenance; Pericardiocentesis.; Management of Pneumothorax with Needle Insertion/Drainage	
	Privilege Core	Metrics
	Fiberoptic Bronchoscopy, Dx and Tx	Volume, Clinical Outcomes, Efficiency, Processes of Care, Reviews
	ET Intubation, Including Airway Maintenance	Volume, Clinical Outcomes, Efficiency, Processes of Care, Reviews
	Insertion of Central Venous, Arterial, and Pulmonary Artery Balloon Flotation Catheters	Volume, Clinical Outcomes, Efficiency, Processes of Care, Reviews
	Management of Pneumothorax with Needle Insertion and Drainage	Volume, Clinical Outcomes, Efficiency, Processes of Care, Reviews
	Pericardiocentesis	Volume, Clinical Outcomes, Efficiency, Processes of Care, Reviews
	Thoracentesis	Volume, Clinical Outcomes, Efficiency, Processes of Care, Reviews
Special	Fluoroscopy	Volume, Clinical Outcomes, Efficiency, Processes of Care, Reviews
	Procedural Sedation	Volume, Clinical Outcomes, Efficiency, Processes of Care, Reviews
	Swan-Canz Catheter Placement	Volume, Clinical Outcomes, Efficiency, Processes of Care, Reviews
	CVP Line Insertion	Volume, Clinical Outcomes, Efficiency, Processes of Care, Reviews
	Rigid Bronchoscopy	Volume, Clinical Outcomes, Efficiency, Processes of Care, Reviews

References: "Yale-New Haven Hospital," 2014.

Table 3.10 Behavioral Health/Psychiatry

Core	**Definition**: AEDTC, and Help Rehabilitate Patients with Behavioral Health Conditions, Chronic and Emergent, and Substance Use/Abuse Conditions. Treatments May include Comprehensive and Intensive Therapeutic Services for Adults with Functional and Organic Psychiatric Disorders, Treating Emergent Symptoms and Preparing Patients to be Treated, in the Future, in a Less Restrictive Environment. **Procedures include**: Evaluate Cognitive/Psychosocial Capability; Determine Baseline Mental/Behavioral Functioning; Evaluate and Establish Impact of Brain Injuries/Disorders on Patient Functional Abilities; Transcranial Magnetic Stimulation; Biofeedback Treatment; Cognitive-Behavioral Therapy; Specialized Disorder Evaluations; Medical Management of Cognitive and Behavioral Challenges/Conditions; Therapy (including Individual, Group, Family, Other); Crisis Intervention; Psychiatric Diagnostic Activities, using DSM; Differential Diagnoses of Patients Presenting with Medical/Neurological Disorders with Behavioral Symptoms	
	Privilege Core	**Metrics**
	Specialized Evaluation	Volume, Clinical Outcomes, Efficiency, Processes of Care, Reviews
	Functional Assessment	Volume, Clinical Outcomes, Efficiency, Processes of Care, Reviews
	Therapy	Volume, Clinical Outcomes, Efficiency, Processes of Care, Reviews
Child and Adolescent Psychiatry	**Definition:** AEDTC, and Help Rehabilitate Patients from Birth to Young Adulthood with Behavioral Health, Cognitive, and/or Developmental Conditions, Chronic or Emergent and Substance Use/Abuse Conditions. **Procedures include:** Clinical Intervention; Mental Status Evaluation; Psychiatric Diagnosis, using DSM; Crisis Intervention; Interpretation of Psychiatric/Psychological Test Results; Diagnose and Management Patients Presenting with Medical/Neurological Disorders with Behavioral Systems; Child Behavioral Management; Identify and Address/Treat Physical, Emotional, and/or Sexual Abuse, Neglect; Evaluate Cognitive Challenges/Conditions	
	Privilege Child/Adolescent Psych	**Metrics**
	Procedures Requiring Transection of the GI Tract	Volume, Clinical Outcomes, Efficiency, Processes of Care, Reviews
	Gastric Banding	Volume, Clinical Outcomes, Efficiency, Processes of Care, Reviews
Chemical Dependency, Addiction Medicine	**Definition**: Assessment, Diagnosis, and Treatment of Substance Use Disorders (Addiction, Abuse, Intoxication, and Withdrawal Disorders); Management of Severe or Complex Intoxication and Withdrawal; Management of Complications of Substance Use Disorders **Procedures include:** Assessment/Diagnosis of Withdrawal, Moderate Withdrawal, and Moderate Intoxication; Assessment/Diagnosis of Addiction and Substance-Use Disorders; Management of Severe/Complex Intoxication/Withdrawal; Management of Medical Complications of Addiction and Other Substance-Use Disorders; Management of Psychiatric Complications of Addiction and Other Substance-Use Disorders; Screening/Referral for Dual Diagnosis (Mental Health Disorder plus Addictive Disorder); Assessment/Management of Dual Diagnosis.	
	Privilege Privilege Chemical Dependency/Addiction	**Metrics**
	Liver Transplant	Volume, Clinical Outcomes, Efficiency, Processes of Care, Reviews
	Kidney-Pancreas	Volume, Clinical Outcomes, Efficiency, Processes of Care, Reviews
Special	ECT	Volume, Clinical Outcomes, Efficiency, Processes of Care, Reviews
	Detoxification for Chemical Dependency	Volume, Clinical Outcomes, Efficiency, Processes of Care, Reviews
	Biofeedback	Volume, Clinical Outcomes, Efficiency, Processes of Care, Reviews

References: "Hospital-based psychiatric," 2014; "Delineation of privileges for child psychiatry." 2014; "Detroit Medical Center," 2009; "Clinical privilege white paper," 2012.

Table 3.11 Rehabilitation/Physical Medicine

Core	**Definition**: Treat Patients of All Ages with Physical Impairments and/or Disabilities involving Neuromuscular, Neurologic, Cardiovascular, or Musculoskeletal Disorders; includes Treatment of Uncomplicated Cardiovascular, Gastrointestinal, Genitourinary, and Respiratory Tract Diseases, and Uncomplicated Skin Programs (e.g., Pressure Ulcers and Abscesses). May include Physical Examination and Development of Treatment Plans for Pain/Weakness/Numbness Syndromes, Using Physical Agents and Interventions. **Procedures include:** Application of Orthotic Materials; Anesthetic and/or Motor Blocks; Arthrocentesis and Joint Injection; Disability Evaluations; Ergonomic Evaluations; Fitness for Duty Evaluations; Joint Manipulation and Mobilization; Prescription of Orthotics, Prosthetics, Wheelchairs, and Adaptive Equipment	
	Privilege Core	Metrics
	Fitness for Duty Evaluations	Volume, Clinical Outcomes, Efficiency, Processes of Care, Reviews
	Arthrocentesis	Volume, Clinical Outcomes, Efficiency, Processes of Care, Reviews
	Ergonomic Evaluations	Volume, Clinical Outcomes, Efficiency, Processes of Care, Reviews
Brain Injury Medicine	**Definition:** Focused on the Prevention, Evaluation, Treatment, and Rehabilitation of Patients who Have an Acquired Brain Injury **Procedures List:** Evaluation of Cognitive Functioning; Fitness to Drive Assessments; Neuropsychiatric Assessments; Monitoring of Function via Simulation	
	Privilege Brain Injury	Metrics
	Evaluation of Cognitive Functioning	Volume, Clinical Outcomes, Efficiency, Processes of Care, Reviews
	Fitness to Drive Assessments	Volume, Clinical Outcomes, Efficiency, Processes of Care, Reviews
	Neuropsychiatric Assessments	Volume, Clinical Outcomes, Efficiency, Processes of Care, Reviews
Pain Medicine	**Definition**: Diagnoses and Treats Patients Experiencing Acute, Chronic, and/or Cancer Pain in the Hospital Setting. **Procedures include:** Peripheral Nerve Blocks; Joint and Bursal Sac Injections; Electrical Stimulation; Implantation/Monitoring of Epidural and Intrathecal Catheters, Ports, and Infusion Pumps; Cryotherapeutic Techniques	
	Privilege Pain Medicine	Metrics
	Peripheral Nerve Blocks	Volume, Clinical Outcomes, Efficiency, Processes of Care, Reviews
	Joint Injections	Volume, Clinical Outcomes, Efficiency, Processes of Care, Reviews
	Electrical Stimulation	Volume, Clinical Outcomes, Efficiency, Processes of Care, Reviews
Special	Venipuncture	Volume, Clinical Outcomes, Efficiency, Processes of Care, Reviews
	Hypnosis, Stress Management, and Relaxation	Volume, Clinical Outcomes, Efficiency, Processes of Care, Reviews
	Trigeminal Ganglionectomy	Volume, Clinical Outcomes, Efficiency, Processes of Care, Reviews

References: *"Physical medicine and rehabilitation," 2013; Yale, Honsotia, Knapp, & Ehrfurth, 2003; "Huntington Hospital, delineation of privileges," 2014*

NOTES

Chapter 4

Preparing Special Meals:
Profiling Pathology, Radiology, Emergency
Medicine, and Anesthesiology

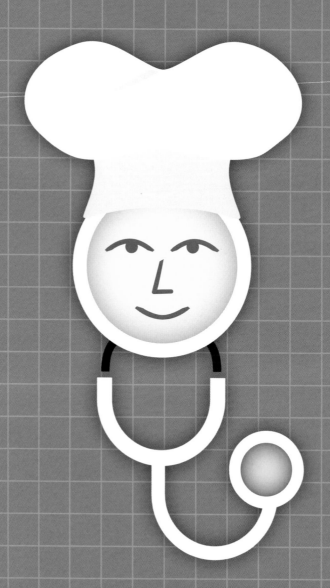

The Kitchen Is Busy...

At times, special groups come to dinner, and you need to create custom menus to meet their needs. Consider some of your most important guests with unique tastes: Pathology, Radiology, Emergency Medicine, and Anesthesiology. Be sure to talk to these diners in advance to see what they need and what they really want!

Next, work with them to build the menu, and then go looking for the correct ingredients.

Warning: you may have to shop at some specialty stores to find the right items – most supermarkets don't stock what you will need for this crowd!

We have covered the majority of hospital providers with inpatient privileges – Internists, Hospitalists, Pediatricians, and Surgeons whose clinical activities for inpatients can be categorized by provider status as Admitting, Attending, Consultant, or Procedure Provider. As we have seen, solid profiles for these providers can be created from a robust discharge dataset. However, there are 4 high volume specialties that are an essential part of all hospitals that are not readily profiled by discharge datasets, and whose services are somewhat different than the majority of the Medical Staff: Pathology, Radiology, Emergency Medicine, and Anesthesiology. We have nicknamed these "the Big Four."

Of the Big Four, 3 (Pathology, Radiology, and Emergency Medicine) share a key characteristic - reaching a diagnosis as quickly and accurately as possible. While Emergency providers also provide essential treatment in the Emergency Room, their care is generally designed to begin treatment that will be continued by others, either on an inpatient or outpatient basis. So for these 3, quality metrics tend to emphasize throughput Efficiency by measuring time intervals between defined benchmark events[1], as well as the Accuracy of diagnosis. In addition to these metrics, it is important to profile providers by the privileges that they have within their departments.

---

[1] For example, consider the following: ED Arrival to Treatment Space Time, Treatment Space to Provider Time, Arrival to Provider Time [aka "door to doc"], ED Length of Stay, Laboratory Test Turn-Around Time, Waiting Time in Radiology, Time from Image Capture to Interpretation.

Rather than trying to provide a sample profile by department, let's look at each of these 3 departments with this commonality in mind, and consider the resources that can help create robust provider profiles for these specialties. See Table 4.1, where our major domains used in the prior chapters are listed, with reference to these 3 specialties.

Table 4.1 Pathology, Radiology, Emergency Medicine draft

DOMAIN	PATHOLOGY	RADIOLOGY	EMERGENCY MEDICINE
Volume	Volume by Cases, Case Types, Clinical and Anatomic	Volume by Case Types; Interventional Volume	Number of ED Encounters by Time
Acuity			See Benchmarking Summit: ESI/CTAS, or E and M Codes
Outcome (including Accuracy of Diagnosis)	Results of Double Reads/Over Reads, Laboratory Proficiency Testing	Results of Double Reads/Over Reads	Morality Rates; Complications of Procedures; % of ED Outpatients Admitted as Inpatients (Non ICU and ICU); Correlations, Review of Returns to ED within 24-72 Hours; Film and Echo Double Reads
Efficiency	Turnaround Times (TAT), including Time to Frozen Section Reading, Stat Lab, Routine Pathology, Cytology, etc.	Wait Times, Time from Procedure to Reading, Internal Cycle Times	Time Stamps and Interval Metrics; Sub-Cycle Intervals; CMS ED Core Measures; Utilization; Emergency Service Units; Door to Provider, etc. (Welch, 2006, 2011)
Processes of Care	Turn-Around Times (TAT)	Radiation Dosage Metrics (Especially CT)	Identification, Triage, etc. (Welch, 2011); Core Measures Related to ED Compliance with Guidelines (Sepsis, Chest Pain, etc.)

DOMAIN	PATHOLOGY	RADIOLOGY	EMERGENCY MEDICINE
Privilege-Based Metrics	Clinical Pathology (Immunohematology, Blood Banking, Hematology, Hematopathology, Clinical Microbiology): Proficiency Testing Anatomic Pathology (Surgical, Autopsy, Cytopathology, Molecular): Correlation of Frozen to Final Diagnoses; Results of Double Reading Procedural Services	Special Procedures: Angiography, CT or Ultrasound Guided Needle Biopsy, Other Interventions	Ultrasound
Customer Satisfaction	Survey of Referring Physicians and Staff on Communication, Timeliness, and Accuracy	Communication with Referring Clinician; Patient Satisfaction with Radiology Department	ED CAHPS Survey Left Without Being Seen, Before Treatment Complete, Against Medical Advice; Patient Complaints, Total and Rates
Citizenship	Timely Dictation, Availability when on Call, Meeting Attendance, CME	Timely Dictation; Availability When on Call; Meeting Attendance, CME	Medical Records; Meeting Attendance; Training; On-Time; Missed Shifts
Review	Review of Cases, Triggered by Metrics	Review of Cases, Triggered by Metrics	Review of Cases, Triggered by Metrics

Pathology

Chances are great that your Pathology Department already has a robust quality control program in place, and may already be creating competency reports by provider. The College of American Pathologists (CAP) continues to be very active in both continuing education and laboratory accreditation. In 2009, its Practice Management Committee published a review of the general requirements for Medical Staff privileging and how they apply to Pathologists (Catalano et. al, 2009). The committee identified activities and metrics to address these requirements, and how they can be applied to OPPE and FPPE processes. See Table 4.1, Pathology.

To further this work, CAP introduced a software data product Evalumetrics™ for OPPE and FPPE (Karcher et. al, 2013). Evalumetrics™ is divided into 4 major categories:

1. General Pathology, including metrics applicable to all Pathologists such as continuing education and on-call performance
2. Clinical Pathology, including immunohematology, blood banking, hematology, hematopathology, and clinical microbiology
3. Anatomic Pathology, including surgical pathology, autopsy pathology, cytopathology, and molecular pathology
4. Procedural Services

The Evalumetrics™ methodology recognizes 3 major areas of performance: practice activity (Volume); timeliness; and competence, with an emphasis on review of both cases and comparative data by peers (Karchner et. al, 2013).

When developing Pathology profiles, focus on the privileges that each Pathology provider has and look for metrics that will reflect performance in these areas. Remember that Pathology is special in that the providers not only provide a professional service, but also run an essential hospital department, including programs for quality, safety, and performance improvement.

Radiology

Radiology is similar to Pathology in that its providers work together in an integrated department of the hospital that is typically under contract to provide services. Provider performance centers on the Accuracy and Precision of reading and interpreting diagnostic images, as well as providing interventional services under radiographic guidance, a service that has grown in recent years.

While Volume by Privilege continues to be important, additional metrics may include: Waiting Times for Studies, Turn-Around Times for Reports, Interpretation of Studies in Light of the Patient's Clinical Status, and Communication with the Care Team. In addition, Double Reading of a sample of studies has been the backbone of internal quality measurement for many years, with desired correlation targets of >90 percent (Steele et. al, 2010).

Much of the double-reading (also referred to as "over-reading") peer review is now managed electronically, either locally or through national peer review datasets. With the advent of digital imaging and Picture Archiving and Communication Systems (PACS), radiographic image capture, reading, and storage is now electronic. Many of these systems provide random selection of cases for Double Reading, providing a Radiologist a certain number of repeat readings during an average work day, then aggregating these results for purposes of provider profiling.

On a national level, the American College of Radiology established a task force on patient safety in 2000 in response to the 1999 IOM report "To Err is Human: Building a Safer Health System" ("To Err is," 1999). One of the ACR committees addressed model peer review and self-evaluation, developing the RADPEER™ program, a Radiology peer-review process. Following a 14 site pilot trial, the program was offered to ACR members in 2002 (Jackson et. al, 2009; Larson et. al, 2009). RADPEER™ is a web-based system which provides confidential peer review of studies in departments for a size-based department fee, providing confidential reports to department heads. As of 2010, more than 10,000 Radiologists and 800 practice groups had participated (Steele, 2010).

Finally, safety in Radiology services continues to be a critical issue; elements that may be included in this area run the gamut, from assuring that the right patient gets the right study, that all positive findings are appropriately communicated to the care team, and that radiation dosage, both by test and by patient, is within acceptable limits. The last of these has become a more prominent issue in recent years as rapid CT scanning for emergent conditions, such as Stroke, has been developed, often requiring higher dosage per test, as well as repeat testing. Consider metrics on dosage for department-level reporting at first, then broken down by provider, as applicable.

Emergency Medicine

Emergency Services provide timely care to treat emergency conditions, save life and limb, and alleviate suffering, based on an accurate diagnosis. Similar to Pathology and Radiology, a large part of service measurement in this department involves creating time stamps at key points during the patient's stay, and measuring the intervals between these times. Other measures include determining the Accuracy of Diagnoses and the Appropriateness of Treatment.

Toward these ends, an Emergency Medicine collaborative on benchmarking met in 2006 and 2010, creating consensus on Emergency Department operational metrics, measures, and definitions (Welch et. al, 2006, 2011). Its objectives were to develop a core set of metrics for ED patient flow and operations; define the metrics clearly using timestamps, time intervals, and proportions; and standardize the vocabulary relevant to the practice of Emergency Medicine operations, including operating characteristics, processes, and utilization. We have summarized some of these in Table 4.1, but encourage the reader to review the original publications.

Additional work in the area of Quality and Outcomes for Emergency Care was published in 2002 by Patrice Lindsay et al., reporting results of an expert panel Modified-Delphi process used to identify specific condition-outcome pairs where there is an identified link between quality of care for the condition and a specific outcome. The panel identified 8 disease-specific process-outcome pairs (asthma, pneumonia, acute myocardial infarction, deep vein thrombosis/pulmonary embolism, chest pain, minor head trauma, and ankle trauma); with the exception of minor head trauma, all were then associated with specific indicators paired to the outcomes of Mortality, Morbidity, Return to ED, Diagnostic Testing, and Admission. Of interest to those developing provider profiles is that many of these indicators involve Time Intervals between defined time stamps (Lindsay et. al, 2002).

In the same issue of *Academic Emergency Medicine*, Graff and colleagues. presented findings of another consensus committee on how quality in Emergency Medicine can be measured and how quality improvement projects can positively impact the care of Emergency patients. This review provides sample measures for disease-specific conditions, including Acute Myocardial Infarction, Pneumonia, Asthma, and Heart Failure, as well as a range of diagnostic syndromes (Graff et. al, 2002).

Starting with the above as guidelines, work with your Emergency Department providers to find meaningful metrics that fit the population served and the department workflow.

Anesthesiology

Unlike Pathology, Radiology, and Emergency Medicine, Anesthesiology is a specialty that provides specific services of Anesthesia and Pain Management for patients under the primary care of a Surgeon or Internist. Although rapid diagnosis of events while under Anesthesia is an essential attribute of the specialty, the bulk of the work is routine; measures tend to center on internal (peer) and external (patient) satisfaction with services, as well as Safety and Efficiency.

Using the TQ profile configuration, with mapping to ACGME, a draft profile for Anesthesiology is provided in Table 4.2. The measures are similar to those for other providers, including Volume, Process and Outcomes Overall and by Privilege. In alignment with our approach in Chapter 3, the privilege-based measures should draw their structure from the Medical Staff privileging process. A well-defined core privileging system will help direct and define the metrics for this profile.

The biggest challenge for Anesthesia is the identification of data sources. Approximately 70 percent of all anesthetics today are used in association with ambulatory patients – either hospital outpatients or in surgery centers, offices, and clinics. Estimates for "Non-Operating Room Anesthesia" range from 30 to 50 percent of all cases in most university practices (Richard Dutton, personal communication; October 2, 2014). Therefore, the first place to look for data is the IT system that is common for all procedures regardless of location: the billing system. Most Anesthesia billing systems include cases by CPT code, with case type, and time of procedure.

Secondary data sources include operating room datasets or Anesthesia information management systems (AIMS), the latter serving as electronic medical records for Operating Room Anesthesia cases.

Although AIMS solutions have been in use for more than 20 years (Stonemetz & Ruskin, 2009), usage has grown in the past 5 years in response to meaningful use incentives and the rise of electronic medical records. However, they will only capture data from OR cases, and miss provider cases performed outside of the OR. For more information on how these systems can be used for profiling, see a recent report from the Massachusetts General Hospital (Ehrenfeld et. al, 2012) and the book *Anesthesia Informatics* (Stonemetz & Ruskin, 2009).

Another good resource is the National Anesthesia Clinical Outcomes Registry (NACOR), a voluntary professional database maintained by the Anesthesia Quality Institute (AQI), which provides OPPE and benchmarking services for anesthesia providers. NACOR has been designated as a Qualified Clinical Data Registry (QCDR) by CMS for Physician Quality Reporting System (PQRS) reporting. The registry provides participating providers peer-to-peer benchmarks, as well as custom continuous performance monitors, performance gap analysis, patient outlier identification, and access to improvement interventions ("National anesthesia clinical," 2014). The registry included over 22 million cases as of January 2015, with participation by 25 percent of providers in the United States (Richard Dutton, personal communication, 2015).

AQI also runs the Anesthesia Incident Reporting System (AIRS), an AHRQ listed Patient Safety Organization (PSO), which supports confidential reporting of anesthesia events with the protections of the Patient Safety and Quality Improvement Act of 2005. AIRS includes 4 sub-specialty modules based on common event types: Respiratory Depression, Drug Shortage, Obstetrics, and Pediatrics ("Anesthesia Incident Reporting System," 2015).

Finally, a comment on the growing use of simulation training, both in residency programs and for established providers. Simulation training can be extremely helpful, especially for specialties where team management of time critical events is important, such as Anesthesiology. Consider adding simulation training to your CME program, and recording participation in your profiles ("Simulation education," 2015).

Procedural Sedation

We are including this topic as a separate heading, but under the general rubric of Anesthesia. Procedural sedation is a major activity in most hospitals, and a potential source of complications. The Director of Anesthesia is generally in charge of sedation institution-wide, including responsibility for credentialing, training, policies, and quality management, regardless of the specialty of the practitioner providing the sedation. In Chapter 3, Procedural Sedation is commonly listed as a special privilege for the certain specialties, among them Gastroenterology, as well as Radiology and Emergency Medicine. The Anesthesia Quality Institute provides excellent recommendations for quality metrics for Procedural Sedation, which can be used as part of profiling for all providers with these privileges, see Appendix 4.1

Summary

In this chapter, we have addressed provider profiling for the 4 specialties that are not easily measured with commonly available administrative datasets. Now that we have added profiles for Pathology, Radiology, Emergency Medicine, and Anesthesiology, we have covered a majority of Medical Staff members with privileges. Next, we need to address profiles for non-physician providers, Advanced Practice Clinicians.

Reference List:

"Anesthesia Incident Reporting System." (2014). Retrieved from http://aqihq.org/airsIntro.aspx

Catalano E.D., Ruby S.G., Talbert M.L., & Knapman D.G. (2009). College of American Pathologists considerations for the delineation of pathology clinical privileges. *Arch Pathol Lab Med*, (133), 613-618.

Ehrenfeld, J.M., Henneman, J.P., Peterfreund, R.A., Sheehan, T.D., Xue, F., Spring, S., & Sandberg, W.S. (2012). Ongoing Professional Performance Evaluation (OPPE) using automatically captured electronic anesthesia data. *The Joint Commission Journal on Quality and Patient Safety*, (38), 73-80.

Graff, L., Stevens, C., Spaite, D., & Foody, J. (2002) Measuring and improving quality in emergency medicine. *Academy of Emergency Medicine*, (9), 1091-1107.

Jackson, V.P., Cushing, T., Abujudeh, H.H., Borgstede, J.P., Chin, K.W., Grimes, C.H., …Thorwath, W.T. (2009). RADPEER scoring white paper. *Journal of the American College of Radiology*, (6), 21-25.

Karcher, D., Howanitz, P.J., Nakhleh, R.E., & Schifman, R.B. (2013). Evalumetrics™ for pathologists' ongoing professional practice evaluation (OPPE) and focused professional practice evaluation (FPPE). *College of American Pathologists White Paper* (2).

Larson, P.A., Pyatt, R.S., Grimes, C.K., Abudujeh, H.H., Chin, K.W., & Roth, C.J. (2011). Getting the most out of RADPEER. *Journal of the American College of Radiology*, (8), 543-548.

Lindsay, P., Schull, M., Bronskill, S., & Anderson, G. (2002). The development of indicators to measure the quality of clinical care in emergency departments following a modified-Delphi approach. *Academy of Emergency Medicine*, (9), 1131-1139.

"National Anesthesia Clinical Outcomes Registry." (2014). Anesthesia Quality Institute. Retrieved from http://aqihq.org/introduction-to-nacor.aspx

"Quality Metrics for Procedural Sedation." (2015) Anesthesia Quality Institute. Retrieved from www.aqihq.org/files/Procedural_Sedation_Metrics.docx

"Simulation education network." (2015). Retrieved from https://www.asahq.org/education/simulation-education

Steele, J.R., Hovsepian, D.M., & Schomer, D.F. (2010) The Joint Commission practice performance evaluation: A primer for radiologists. *Journal of the American College of Radiology*, (7), 425-430.

Stonemetz, J., & Ruskin, K., Ed. (2009). *Anesthesia Informatics*. London: Springer-Verlag London Limited

"To Err is Human: Building a Safer Health System." (1999). Institute of Medicine, National Academy of Health. Retrieved from https://www.iom.edu/~/media/Files/Report%20Files/1999/To-Err-is-Human/To%20Err%20is%20Human%20 1999%20%20report%20brief.pdf

Welch, S., Augustine, J., Camargo, C.A., & Reese, C. (2006). Emergency department performance measures and benchmarking summit. *Academic Emergency Medicine*, (13), 1074-1080.

Welch, S.J., Asplin, B.R., Stone-Griffith, S., Davidson, S.J., Augustine, J., & Schuur, J. (2011). Emergency department operational metrics, measures and definitions: Results of the second performance measures and benchmarking summit. *Academic Emergency Medicine*, (58:1), 33-40.

NOTES

Appendix 4.1
Quality Metrics for Procedural Sedation, Anesthesia Quality Institute

Quality Metrics for Procedural Sedation

AQI consensus recommendations for the Director of Anesthesia Services charged with initiating a quality management program in procedural sedation. Data must be gathered each month from each unit where patients receive sedation. Data gathering should be modified as necessary to fit the information technology available and the patient population served.

Core Elements

Volume Metrics
- Type and number of procedures performed
- Number of patients receiving light or moderate sedation
    - Number receiving sedation via Computer-Assisted Personalized Sedation (CAPS)
- Number of patients receiving deep sedation
- Number of patients cared for by an anesthesia team

Outcomes
- Cases completed as planned, without complication, versus:
- Cases cancelled due to patient discomfort or anxiety
- Cases with unplanned escalation in the continuum of sedation
- Patients receiving rescue medication: flumazenil or naloxone
- Unplanned respiratory support required in light or moderate sedation cases
    - Placement of nasal trumpet or oral airway
    - Placement of supraglottic airway (e.g. LMA) or endotracheal tube
    - Assisted ventilation with bag-valve-mask
    - Oxygen saturation < 85 percent for greater than 3 minutes
- Patients experiencing a serious adverse event (e.g. perforation, anaphylaxis, cardiac arrest)
- Unplanned admission of an outpatient within 24 hours
- Unplanned patient transfer to an Emergency Department

Optional Elements

As the quality program matures and information technology capabilities advance, these data will enable further improvements in patient care:

- Patient demographics: age, sex, ASA Physical Status
- Procedure duration
- Medications used: doses and times
- PACU and facility length of stay
- Patient satisfaction: at PACU discharge and at 48 hours post-procedure
- Provider satisfaction: proceduralist and nursing staff

("Quality Metrics for Procedural Sedation," 2015)

Table 4.2 Anesthesiology

DOMAINS	CATEGORY	ANESTHESIA MEASURE SUMMARY	ACGME
Patient Care	Volume	Volume of Discharges as Attending, Procedures Provider, Consultant Volume of Cases by Types of Anesthesia	Patient Care
Patient Care	Acuity	Volume by ASA Classification and/or Location, Subdivided by Types of Anesthesia	Patient Care
Patient Care	Clinical Outcome	Clinical Outcomes of Care including Mortality, Complications, and Other Events, Risk Adjusted when Possible; Re-intubation within XX Hours Post Anesthesia	Patient Care
Patient Care	Efficiency	On-Time First Case Starts; Turn-Over Time; Same-Day Case Cancellations	Systems-Based Practice
Patient Care	Processes of Care	Core Measures; Compliance with Other Best Practices; Drug and Blood Utilization; Time Out Compliance, by Team; Pre-Anesthesia Assessment Completed; Post-Anesthesia Assessment Completed; Non-Compliance with Standards for Basic Anesthesia Monitoring: Count	Patient Care
Privilege-Based Performance	General Anesthesia, Including Pre- and Post-Operative Treatment	Volume, Acuity, Processes, Clinical Outcomes, and Efficiency Measures	Patient Care, Systems-Based Practice
Privilege-Based Performance	Placement of Arterial and Central Venous Lines	Volume, Acuity, Processes, Clinical Outcomes, and Efficiency Measures	Patient Care, Systems-Based Practice
Privilege-Based Performance	Regional Anesthesia: Spinal, Epidural, and Peripheral Nerve Blocks	Volume, Acuity, Processes, Clinical Outcomes, and Efficiency Measures	Patient Care, Systems-Based Practice
Privilege-Based Performance	Pain Management	Volume, Acuity, Processes, Clinical Outcomes, and Efficiency Measures	Patient Care, Systems-Based Practice
Patient Care	Patient Satisfaction	Results of Patient Satisfaction Surveys Validated Patient Complaints	Interpersonal and Communication Skills

DOMAINS	CATEGORY	ANESTHESIA MEASURE SUMMARY	ACGME
Citizenship	Citizenship	Timely Completion of Medical Records, including Discharge Summaries, Operative Notes, History/Physicals; Compliance with Medical Staff Bylaws, Rules, and Regulations; Internal Staff Surveys and Validated Complaints; Participation in Medical Staff Committees; Participation In-House Officer Training Programs; CME Credits per Quarter; Participation in Simulation Training	Professionalism, Medical Knowledge
Review	Review	Count of All Cases Peer Reviewed, with Outcomes of Reviews; Risk Management Claims Pending and Settled or Pending; Review of Any Issues; Invasive Procedure, Infection Control, Blood Usage, Pharmacy and Therapeutics	Practice-Based Learning and Improvement

NOTES

NOTES

Chapter 5

Planning for New Dinner Guests: Advanced Practice Clinicians

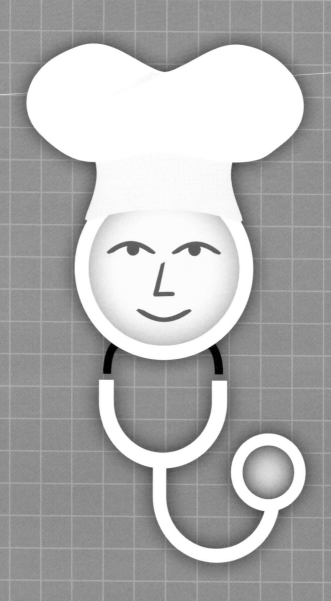

Our Work Continues...

Now that you have experience with custom menus for Pathology, Radiology, Emergency Medicine, and Anesthesiology, it's time to get ready for a new crowd, Advanced Practice Clinicians (APCs)!

APCs sit at the table with everyone else, but need a special blend of unique ingredients, prepared in a special way that matches their unique roles as independent providers, often working in partnership with physicians in the care of patients. As with the Big 4 covered in the previous chapter, data for APCs comes from custom datasets that capture their activity accurately.

Here is your chance to be creative in order to most effectively meet this group's needs. But, as always, it's important that you work closely with your diners to deliver the meals they want and need.

As discussed in the Introduction, professional practice profiles need to be created not just for physicians, but also for Advanced Practice Clinicians (APCs). These include those professional providers who are not physicians, but work with physicians to care for patients in most of the environments where a physician provider practices. For the purposes of this discussion, we will group all APCs together; this group includes a varied array of potential members, including Certified Registered Nurse Anesthetists (CRNAs), Certified Nurse Midwives (CNMs), Nurse Practitioners (NPs), and Physician Assistants (PAs). These 4 account for the majority of practicing APCs, though some may assert that there are additional professional practitioners who fit into this group (Weitz, Anderson, & Taylor, 2009).

Note that although we will be referring to these practitioners as APCs, this is not the only way to reference them. For instance, Medicare labels these healthcare professionals as "Non-Physician Practitioners," listing Nurse Practitioners, Clinical Nurse Specialists, and Physician Assistants as the providers who practice collaboratively, or under the supervision of a physician ("Medicare coverage," 2001).

This grouping is very complex and varied; each role could easily fill up its own chapter. Hence, although we cover this group of providers in a single chapter, we have attempted to provide additional information on APCs through this chapter's references. Since the APC field has seen rapid growth in the past 30 years, regulatory agencies require ongoing evaluation of their performance; more hospitals are profiling these non-physician providers who care for their patient populations, in both inpatient and outpatient settings.

Your hospital organization may already have a profiling process established for APCs, but this evolving area is continually growing and improving; therefore, we provide our recommendations for building profiles in the following pages.

We will explore the 4 identified primary subsets of APCs, and provide information on typical privilege sets, as well as a draft set of sample indicators for each subset. We hope these drafts will serve as a starting place as you further develop your APC profiles. As with other information shared throughout this text, we want to remind you that our offerings are a starting point; you will certainly need to revise and edit our content so that you are able to meet your organization's needs. Recall that "no drafts are perfect, but all drafts are helpful." See Chapter 1 for more information.

Certified Registered Nurse Anesthetist (CRNA)

The first sub-category of professionals who fall into the grouping of APC is the Certified Registered Nurse Anesthetist (CRNA). With ties to the 1860s during the American Civil War, Nurses provided Anesthesia to soldiers wounded in battle. The formal introduction of Nurse Anesthesia to academia in the United States was in 1909 at St. Vincent's Hospital in Portland, Oregon. The Certified Registered Nurse Anesthetist credential came into existence much later, however. It was not until 1956 that a nurse providing Anesthesia care to Surgical, Obstetrical, Pain Management, and Trauma patients could achieve this deemed level of expertise ("History of nurse anesthesia," 2010).

The CRNA is vital in hospitals across the nation, with Anesthesia professionals administering more than 34 million Anesthetics to patients yearly, per the AANA's 2013 Practice Profile Survey. In rural America in particular, CRNAs are the primary providers of Anesthesia Care; in this role, they allow non-urban hospitals to offer high quality, comprehensive care to patients within the hospital environment. Working in cohort with Surgeons,

Anesthesiologists, Dentists, Podiatrists, and other healthcare professionals, CRNAs practice in a very autonomous way, as illustrated by the fact that legislation passed by Congress in 1986 made Nurse Anesthetists the first nursing specialty to be accorded direct reimbursement rights under Medicare ("Certified registered nurse," 2015).

The CRNA's scope of practice varies from state to state. In some states, a collaborative relationship between a supervising physician and the CRNA is required; in these states, the Nurse Anesthetist is the responsibility of the physician and receives medical direction from him/her. In other states, the CRNA must have consent from the physician to administer the Anesthesia. And in still others, the CRNA is able to act independently, making clinical judgments based on his or her own knowledge and recognized skill set (Malina & Izlar, 2014).

The CRNA is authorized to deliver comprehensive Anesthesia Care under each state's Nurse Practice Act. This authorization includes all accepted Anesthesia techniques, including General, Epidural, Spinal, Sedation, and Local. Clinical privileges further define the scope of accepted practice for the CRNA; core privileges may be granted to the CRNA, with details on his/her ability to perform these, as well as more advanced privileges, with or without supervision ("Questions and answers," 2015).

When considering the CRNA scope of practice, it's important to remember that a CRNA is a Registered Nurse. He or she has taken graduate coursework focused on clinical judgment and clinical thinking skills, supporting his/her ability to make informed decisions about Anesthesia Care based on education, licensure, and certification. In the hospital setting, a CRNA provides Anesthesia and Anesthesia-Related Care upon request, assignment, or referral. This professional is tasked with pre-anesthesia preparation and assessment, developing and implementing an Anesthesia plan, initiating General, Local, or Regional Anesthesia or Sedation, monitoring the patient's status, managing the Anesthesia, and maintaining the patient's airway. In addition, the CRNA works to ensure appropriate and healthy emergence from Anesthesia, discharging the patient from Anesthesia Care, managing acute and chronic pain, and responding to emergency situations related to airway management, the use of emergency fluids and drugs, and the provision of Advanced Cardiac Life Support ("CRNA scope of practice," 2014).

See Table 5.1 (p. 142) for Potential CRNA core hospital privileges. We offer this list as an example for reference. The scope of privileges at your hospital will be determined by your state, hospital, and Medical Staff policy. In Table 5.1 (p. 142), the included core privileges have been placed in broad categories, including Anesthesia, Before Use; Anesthesia, Use; Anesthesia, Recovery; Emergency Response; Appropriate Patient Care; Pain Management; and Airway Management.

Remember that the listing of potential special privileges for your CRNAs (included in Table 5.2 (p. 143) should be modified and revised to meet your hospital's needs. It is intended to be a starting point should you need to address your CRNA special privileges.

Once you have a clear list of privileges for CRNAs, you can begin to build metrics for their Professional Practice Profile. Example indicators that may be appropriate to include are listed in Table 5.3, below. Focus on high volume, high risk, and problem-prone areas. Remember that the goal of OPPE is to determine if the provider's performance is adequate to maintain each privilege.

Table 5.3 CRNA Profile draft

INDICATOR/MEASURE	ACGME CATEGORY	TQ DOMAIN
Complete and Accurate Documentation, including Patient Consent Forms	Professionalism; Patient Care	Citizenship
Average CMI of Patient Population	Acuity	Acuity
Rate of Transfer to Patient Care to Anesthesiologist/Other Physician; Communication with Anesthesiologist/Other Physician	Practice-Based Learning and Improvement; interpersonal and Communication	Clinical Outcomes; Privilege-Based Metrics
Patient ALOS (if Identified as Attributed Provider)	Systems-Based Practice	Efficiency
Readmission Rates (if Identified as Attributed Provider)	Systems-Based Practice	Efficiency; Clinical Outcomes
Safety Events (Number and Rate) Related to Anesthesia Plan/Use	Patient Care; Practice-Based Learning and Improvement	Clinical Outcomes; Processes of Care

INDICATOR/MEASURE	ACGME CATEGORY	TQ DOMAIN
Adjusted Cost per Case (if Identified as Attributed Provider)	Systems-Based Practice	Efficiency
Compliance Rate with Policies Relative to the Use of Anesthesia	Patient Care; Practice-Based Learning and Improvement	Citizenship; Processes of Care
Compliance Rate with Policies Relative to the Use of Narcotics and Controlled Substances	Patient Care; Practice-Based Learning and Improvement	Citizenship; Processes of Care
Compliance Rate with Policies Relative to the Use of Blood and Blood Products	Systems-Based Practice; Patient Care; Medical Knowledge	Citizenship; Processes of Care
Patient Complaints (Number and Rate) with Anesthesia Care/Experience (if Identified as Attributed Provider)	Patient Care; Professionalism; Interpersonal and Communication	Patient Satisfaction
Maintenance of Certifications/ Recent Trainings; CME Activity	Practice-Based Learning and Improvement; Medical Knowledge	Citizenship
Antibiotics Given per SCIP Protocols (Rate)	Medical Knowledge	Processes of Care
Appropriate Monitoring Devices Used (Rate)	Medical Knowledge	Processes of Care
Adverse Outcomes/ Complications of Anesthesia, Pain Management Actions, Blood Utilization (Number and Rate)	Medical and Clinical Knowledge; Patient Care; Professionalism	Clinical Outcomes; Processes of Care
Significant Adverse Outcomes/ Complications of Anesthesia, Pain Management Actions, Blood Utilization (Number and Rate)	Medical and Clinical Knowledge; Patient Care; Professionalism	Clinical Outcomes; Processes of Care; Review
Peer Reviewed Cases (if Identified as Attributed Provider; if Identified as Involved Provider)	Practice-Based Learning and Improvement	Review
Internal Satisfaction Surveys	Interpersonal and Communication	Citizenship

If your hospital's CNRA privilege sets change, you will want to include these changes in your privilege-based metrics to ensure you are reviewing each provider in the most comprehensive, appropriate manner.

Finally, let's consider some of the challenges in creating CRNA profiles. Your hospital administrative dataset likely does not identify CRNAs in any of the standard data fields: Admitting, Attending, Principal Procedure, or Discharging Provider. However, you do need to evaluate your CRNAs on metrics associated with Volume, Acuity, and Outcomes. So, look for other data sources to help create these measures. See Chapter 4, where we explore Anesthesia as a specialty area in detail. There, you will find a wide range of potential metrics that may be appropriate not just for your Anesthesiologists' profiles, but also those of your CRNAs. In addition, note that billing data sets may provide you with a great deal of Anesthesia metrics, and have the advantage of covering all locations where Anesthesia or Sedation is employed.

Midwives

Midwives are our second of the 4 major subcategories of APCs. Midwifery dates back thousands of years, to a time well before hospitals existed. The care of the mother and child pre-birth is an ancient practice that has been managed by a Midwife or a person in a Midwife role since ancient times (Sadr, 2014). The hospital-based Midwife became formally recognized in the United States in the mid-1920s, with the first education program beginning in 1932 ("Certified nurse-midwife," 2014).

In the U.S., there are 3 levels of Midwife, most of whom have received training up to or beyond the graduate level. First is the Certified Professional Midwife (CPM). The CPM is the most recent of the Midwife credentials, introduced in the 1980s. Initially issued by the North American Registry of Midwives (NARM) in 1994 ("What is a midwife?", 2014), this credential is intended for practitioners who specialize in child birth outside of the hospital setting; a CPM may not, and often does not, have the Registered Nurse (RN) credential in advance of earning the CPM designation.

The second and smallest of the Midwife roles is the Certified Midwife (CM). This is a practitioner who has studied in a health-related field other than Nursing, and gone on to earn a graduate education from a Midwifery education program accredited by the Accreditation Commission for Midwifery Education (ACME). These providers are not required to have a Nursing background or credential, and most often also perform their duties outside of the hospital ("Types of midwives," 2014).

The third and final role is the Certified Nurse Midwife (CNM). The CNM has the Registered Nurse credential and performs clinical duties outside of the supervision of a physician. CNMs are licensed to perform many of the perinatal services that traditionally fall within the OB/GYN scope of practice. In addition, CNMs today are trained to address most other issues related to family planning and gynecological needs for women of all ages. In many cases, the OB/GYN physician consults on cases that are outside of the CNM's areas of expertise, which may include high-risk pregnancies, or pregnancies in which the mother has a chronic illness or ailment that poses risk to the unborn child ("Certified nurse-midwife," 2013). The CNM is the only of the 3 roles that has authority to write prescriptions in some states.

The CNM credential indicates that the professional has been trained in both nursing and Midwifery, with a focus on providing care within the hospital setting. Further, these practitioners have completed an accredited university-affiliated Nurse-Midwife program, as deemed by the American College of Nurse Midwives; they may be licensed in all states, practicing primarily in hospitals and birth centers ("Frequently asked questions," 2015).

In terms of practice and privileges in the hospital, states vary as to what they allow Certified Nurse Midwives to actually do. For instance, in Alabama (at the time of this writing), CNMs are licensed as Advanced Practice Registered Nurses, and are required to submit a 'collaborative practice agreement' with the physician who will be supervising him or her. Likewise, a CNM practicing in Alabama may request prescribing authority for non-controlled substance medications and drugs ("State by state," 2014).

In Arizona (at the time of this writing), CNMs act as Advanced Registered Nurse Practitioners, must have graduate degrees, and are re-certified every 5 years by the American Midwifery Certification Board (AMCB); within the state, the vast majority of the 206 CNMs registered as of this writing work in hospitals (96%), practicing quite independently ("Midwife licensing," 2014).

When considering hospital privileges that may be granted to a Midwife, the focus is primarily on CNMs; they are, in many situations, the Midwife group with the greatest ability to care for patients independently. Privileges include, but are not limited to, the independent management of women's health care, focusing on pregnancy (including oligohydramnios), childbirth, the postpartum period, care of the newborn, family planning, and gynecological needs of women. Scope of practice may include preconception care, care of the child-bearing woman, health promotion and disease prevention, management of common health problems, and management of peri-menopause and post-menopause. Within a hospital, the CNM may participate in the management of the care of the child-bearing woman who falls into certain potential risk categories in collaboration with a physician consultant. Practice may include admission to and discharge from the hospital and completion of a history and physical. Further, CNMs may provide consultation for well-woman gynecological care to patients who are in the hospital receiving other medical services. In many states, CNMs may write prescriptions appropriate to their scope of practice, and may consult with, collaborate with, or refer within the hospital/system ("Definition of midwifery," 2011).

Table 5.4 (p. 144) illustrates a potential set of core privileges associated with a CNM and is provided for reference. Additional privileges, beyond the core delineated, may be granted to those CNMs who meet qualifications and standards. Table 5.6 (p. 145) lists potential special privileges that may fall into this category. Note that the privileges have been categorized into the following: Post-Birth Patient Care, General Patient Care, Birth Management, Specialized Patient Care, and Infant Care.

Once privileges are outlined for your CNMs, you can move on to consider the metrics that should be included in a profile for this group of providers. The following table offers a starting point for the indicators that may be appropriate for inclusion. Once again, we suggest that you focus on areas that are high volume, high risk, and/or problem-prone. The metrics outlined in Table 5.5 are categorized per both ACGME and the TQ profiling format.

Table 5.5 CNM Profile draft

INDICATOR/MEASURE	ACGME CATEGORY	TQ DOMAIN
Perineal Trauma (Number and Rate)	Patient Care; Acuity; Volume	Clinical Outcomes
Epidurals (Number and Rate)	Patient Care; Acuity; Volume	Volume; Privilege-Based Metrics
Inductions, Elective versus Mandated (Number and Rate)	Patient Care; Acuity; Volume	Volume; Privilege-Based Metrics
Total % of Vaginal Births (Rate)	Patient Care; Volume	Processes of Care; Volume; Privilege-Based Metrics
Total % of Primary C-Sections (if Identified as Attributed Provider; or if Collaborating Care)	Patient Care; Volume	Processes of Care; Volume; Privilege-Based Metrics
Percent of Birth Canal Intact Post Birth	Patient Care	Processes of Care; Clinical Outcomes
%/Rate of Mother Post Birth with Outstanding 3rd or 4th Degree Laceration (if Identified as Attributed Provider)	Patient Care; Acuity; Medical Knowledge	Processes of Care; Clinical Outcomes
Average Gestational Age at Birth	Patient Care; Volume	Process of Care; Volume; Clinical Outcomes
NICU Admissions (Number and Rate)	Patient Care; Acuity	Processes of Care; Clinical Outcomes
Prenatal Visits (Number; Average Number by All Patients)	Patient Care; Volume	Volume
Induction of Labor (Number and Rate), Initiated by a Means Other than Spontaneous Labor but Excluding Augmentation of Labor	Patient Care; Medical Knowledge	Volume; Processes of Care; Privilege-Based Metrics
Total Number of Births	Patient Care; Volume	Volume; Privilege-Based Metrics
Total Number of Full Term Births; Percent of Total Births	Patient Care; Volume	Volume
Total Number of Fetal Deaths; Percent of Total Patients/ Mothers	Patient Care; Volume; Acuity; Medical Knowledge	Clinical Outcomes
Transfer to OB/GYN Physician (Number and Rate)	Systems-Based Practice	Processes of Care; Volume; Clinical Outcomes
Number of Total Births Resulting in a Multiple Birth	Patient Care; Volume; Acuity	Clinical Outcomes

continued >>

125

INDICATOR/MEASURE	ACGME CATEGORY	TQ DOMAIN
Number of Successful Vaginal Births after a Previous Cesarean (VBAC); Number Unsuccessful VBACs (Rate)	Patient Care; Volume; Medical Knowledge	Processes of Care; Volume; Clinical Outcomes
Number of Assisted Vaginal Births (Vacuum Extraction and/or Forceps (Rate)	Patient Care; Volume; Acuity	Processes of Care; Volume; Clinical Outcomes
Number of Episiotomies (Rate)	Patient Care; Volume	Processes of Care; Clinical Outcomes; Privilege-Based Metrics
Infants in Singleton Birth at Less than 37 Weeks Gestation (Rate/Percent)	Practice-Based Learning and Improvement; Volume; Acuity	Processes of Care; Clinical Outcomes; Volume; Acuity
Infants in Singleton Birth Born Weighing Less than 2500 Grams (Rate/Percent)	Practice-Based Learning and Improvement; Volume; Acuity	Processes of Care; Clinical Outcomes; Volume
Birth Mothers Attending 6 Week Postpartum Visit (Rate)	Patient Care; Volume	Processes of Care
Inductions Occurring prior to 41 Weeks Gestational Age (Rate)	Patient Care; Volume	Processes of Care; Clinical Outcomes; Volume
Epidurals Used for Pain Relief During Labor (Including Intrathecals but Excluding Epidural for Sole Purpose of Anesthesia for C-Section or Assisted Vaginal Birth) (Rate)	Patient Care; Volume	Processes of Care; Volume; Clinical Outcomes
Patient Satisfaction with Midwife Care (Rate)	Interpersonal and Communication; Professionalism	Patient Satisfaction
Anesthesia Utilization Rate, by Type	Systems-Based Practice	Processes of Care; Privilege-Based Metrics; Volume
Blood Transfusion Associated with Birth (Number and Rate)	Patient Care; Medical Knowledge	Processes of Care; Privilege-Based Metrics; Volume; Clinical Outcomes
Maternal Death (Number and Rate)	Volume; Acuity	Volume; Clinical Outcomes
Maternal ICU Admission (Number and Rate)	Volume; Acuity	Processes of Care; Volume; Clinical Outcomes
Maternal Return to OR or L&D (Number and Rate)	Volume; Acuity	Processes of Care; Clinical Outcomes; Efficiency
Uterine Rupture (Number and Rate)	Patient Care; Acuity	Processes of Care; Clinical Outcomes
Birth Trauma or Injury (Number and Rate)	Volume; Acuity; Patient Care	Processes of Care; Clinical Outcomes

INDICATOR/MEASURE	ACGME CATEGORY	TQ DOMAIN
Unexpected Admission to Neonatal ICU (>2500 G and Ffr >24 Hr) (Number and Rate)	Volume; Acuity	Processes of Care; Clinical Outcomes
Antenatal Steroids for Under 34 Week Birth (Core Measure PC-03) (Rate)	Medical Knowledge	Processes of Care; Privilege-Based Metrics
Cesarean Rate for Low Risk First Births	Volume; Acuity; Patient Care	Processes of Care; Volume; Privilege-Based Metrics
DVT Prophylaxis for Women Having a C-Section	Volume; Acuity; Patient Care	Processes of Care; Privilege-Based Metrics
Health-Care Associated Bloodstream Infection in Newborns (Core Measure PC-04)	Medical Knowledge; Volume	Processes of Care; Clinical Outcomes
Elective Delivery (at >=37 and < 39 Weeks of Gestation) (Core Measure PC-01)	Medical Knowledge; Volume	Processes of Care; Volume; Privilege-Based Metrics
Provision of Birth Control Education (Number and Rate)	Patient Care; Volume	Processes of Care; Privilege-Based Metrics
Provision of Well Woman Related Exams and Services (Number and Rate)	Patient Care; Medical Knowledge; Volume	Processes of Care; Privilege-Based Metrics
Detection and Appropriate Reporting of Sexual and/or Domestic Violence Situations (Number and Rate)	Patient Care; Medical Knowledge; Volume	Processes of Care; Privilege-Based Metrics
Accurate Diagnosis and Successful Treatment of UTIs, Vaginitis: (Number and Rate)	Medical Knowledge; Patient Care	Privilege-Based Metrics; Clinical Outcomes
CME Activity	Medical Knowledge; Professionalism	Citizenship
Internal Satisfaction Survey Results	Interpersonal and Communication	Citizenship
Adjusted Cost per Case (if Attributed Provider)	Systems-Based Practice	Efficiency
Average CMI of Patient Population	Acuity	Acuity
Peer Reviewed Cases (When Associated with Case; if Attributed Provider)	Practice-Based Learning and Improvement	Reviews
ALOS of Patient Population (if Attributed Provider)	Systems-Based Practice	Efficiency
Readmission Rates (if Attributed Provider)	Systems-Based Practice	Efficiency

If your hospital's CNM privilege sets change, you will want to include these changes in your privilege-based metrics to ensure you are reviewing each provider in the most comprehensive, appropriate manner.

As you consider the measures you wish to include in a profile for CNMs, you will need to address provider attribution, and where you can obtain accurate data. Look toward your hospital and Medical Staff policies in regard to CNM practice, as well as your IT systems in regard to data capture. As noted in the discussion of Anesthesiology and CRNAs, the billing system may be your best source for data on CNM activity.

Nurse Practitioners

As we continue our exploration of APCs, we move next to the Nurse Practitioner (NP). The role of Nurse Practitioner was born of collaborations between Physicians and Nurses in the latter half of the twentieth century ("Mayo School,"2014). The formal Nurse Practitioner role as we may recognize it was developed in 1965, when the University of Colorado offered the first ever NP degree program ("Historical timeline,"2014). Shortly thereafter, many other universities and organizations followed suit. Today, Nurse Practitioners make up just under 200,000 members of the healthcare provider workforce ("All about NPs,"2014).

Educational requirements for Nurse Practitioners vary by state. Given the disparity that exists, contact your state's Department of Health or similar regulatory body for additional information, as needed.

Likewise, the scope of NP practice varies widely from state to state. In some states, including (as of this text's writing) Arizona, New Mexico, Oregon, and Maine, *full practice* is supported. This means that the NP can evaluate, diagnose, order and interpret diagnostic tests, and initiate and manage treatments (including the prescription of medications), under the licensure authority of the state Board of Nursing. This model is recommended by the IOM and by the National Council of State Boards of Nursing ("The future of nursing,"2010).

In other states, including Kansas, Louisiana, and Pennsylvania (at the time of this writing), *reduced practice* is supported. This means that NP clinical activities are limited in at least one significant way. In Pennsylvania, for instance, what is termed "full practice authority" is not supported; instead, within the state, NPs must have a governmentally-mandated contract with a physician in order to practice (Schrand, 2014). Some of these states also require that NPs have a regulated, collaborative agreement with an outside health discipline to provide patient care ("Hospital practice," 2014).

Finally, *restricted practice* is the third possibility, with the most limitations associated with NP practice. States including California, Texas, and Florida (at the time of this writing) allow NPs to practice only with supervision, delegation, or team management by an outside health discipline ("The future of nursing," 2010).

While the details of scope of practice at the state level for a NP differs, in general, the NP scope includes responsibilities associated with Process of Care, care priorities, interdisciplinary and collaborative activities, accurate clinical and patient-related documentation, patient advocacy, quality improvement, and research-based practice (Runyon, 2014).

The required supervision of NPs varies by state; in Missouri, for instance, as of this writing, the 'collaboratory' physician must review 10% of provided care, and 20% of care that includes prescribing, both on a bi-weekly basis ("A guide to understanding," 2014). In addition, some hospital organizations impose additional requirements on the supervision a NP needs in his or her care of patients in the hospital. These requirements range from *General Supervision* to *Direct Supervision* to *Personal Supervision*. Put simply, the first of these, *General Supervision*, requires that the NP be supervised by a Physician, but the Physician does not need to be present while the care is performed. Next, *Direct Supervision* requires that the supervising Physician be available, able to be accessed, and able to provide assistance to the NP as needed. In this case, note that the Physician does not have to be in the same room with the NP when the NP is providing care.

Finally, for *Personal Supervision*, the restrictions are the highest. In this case, the Physician must be in attendance in the room while the care, activity, or procedure is provided or performed (Rhyne, 2008).

You are likely well-informed as to how your team of NPs provide care, and the required supervision associated with their practice. Additional information and aid is available from your state Department of Health and Board of Nursing.

When we consider NP hospital privileges, we are once again able to offer a starting point that may benefit you, should you need to revise or rework your hospital's privilege delineation associated with this APC role. See Table 5.7 (p. 146) for a list of potential core privileges for a NP. Realize that these privileges may be granted within the context of a collaborative management plan with one or more Physicians or Surgeons, as appropriate. Remember, privileges may vary by state. For our organizational purposes, we have grouped the privileges into recommended categories. These include General Patient Care; Quality Improvement; Documentation/Professionalism; Emergency Response; and Specialized Patient Care.

Once core privileges are established, special privileges are next delineated for this group of APCs, the NPs. Potential special privileges that may be granted within your hospital to NPs are listed in Table 5.8 (p. 148). The recommended categories in which these special privileges fall include Specialized Patient Care; General Patient Care: and Patient Care Preparation.

Once privileges are established for the NP, we can move on to determining the metrics that will be used in the profiling of these APCs. In Table 5.9 below, we provide potential indicators that may act as a starting point for your NP profiling metrics. These have been placed in categories associated with our TQ profiling format.

Table 5.9 NP Profile draft

INDICATOR/MEASURE	ACGME CATEGORY	TQ DOMAIN
Complete and Timely Documentation in Medical Record; Compliance (Rate)	Professionalism	Citizenship
Referrals to Supervising Physician or Specialist (Number and Percent)	Volume; Patient Care	Volume; Processes of Care
Appropriate Communication with Medical Team (Rate)	Professionalism	Citizenship
Patient Complaints (Number And Rate)	Professionalism; Patient Care	Patient Satisfaction
Patient Satisfaction; Percent Highly Satisfied or Equivalent	Professionalism; Patient Care	Patient Satisfaction

INDICATOR/MEASURE	ACGME CATEGORY	TQ DOMAIN
Participation in Medical Staff Committees, Projects (Percent or Rate)	Practice-Based Learning and Improvement	Citizenship
Hospital Associated Illness/ Conditions (Number and Rate)	Medical Knowledge; Patient Care; Volume	Processes of Care; Clinical Outcomes
Surgical Site Infections (Number and Rate)	Medical Knowledge; Patient Care	Processes of Care; Clinical Outcomes
Compliance with Discharge Standards (Number and Rate)	Systems-Based Practice	Processes of Care; Volume
Chronic Conditions Management, Identification of Additional Needs (Number and Rate)	Medical Knowledge; Acuity	Processes of Care; Volume
Implementation of Proper Pain/Condition Management Techniques and Monitoring (Number and Rate)	Medical Knowledge	Processes of Care
Blood/Blood Product Utilization (Rate)	Medical Knowledge	Processes of Care
Medication/Rx Utilization (Rate)	Medical Knowledge	Processes of Care
Standard, Best Practice Intervention (Rate)	Medical Knowledge; Practice-Based Learning and Improvement	Processes of Care
Patient Education Plan Compliance (Rate)	Medical; Patient Care	Processes of Care
Patient Evaluation per Standards, Compliance (Rate)	Medical Knowledge; Practice-Based Learning and Improvement	Processes of Care
Diagnostic Testing Appropriate (Rate)	Medical Knowledge	Processes of Care; Clinical Outcomes
Preventative Screening Appropriate (Rate)	Medical Knowledge; Patient Care	Processes of Care; Clinical Outcomes
Participation in In-House Trainings; Maintenance of Certifications and Licensure (Number and Compliance Rate); CME Activity	Practice-Based Learning and Improvement; Medical Knowledge	Citizenship
Achievement of Advanced Clinical Training in Areas of Focus (Number and Percent)	Practice-Based Learning and Improvement; Medical Knowledge	Citizenship
Adjusted Cost per Case (if Attributed Provider)	Systems-Based Practice	Efficiency
Internal Satisfaction Survey Results	Interpersonal and Communication	Citizenship

continued >>

INDICATOR/MEASURE	ACGME CATEGORY	TQ DOMAIN
Peer Reviewed Cases	Practice-Based learning and Improvement	Reviews
ALOS of Patient Population (if Attributed Provider)	Systems-Based Practice	Efficiency
Mortality Rate/Count of Patient Population (if Attributed Provider)	Patient Care	Clinical Outcomes
Average CMI of Patient Population (if Attributed Provider)	Acuity	Acuity

If your hospital's NP privilege sets change, you will want to include these changes in your privilege-based metrics to ensure you are reviewing each provider in the most comprehensive manner.

As with CRNAs and CNMs, attribution and collection of data on clinical activity can be a challenge for this professional category. Work with your leadership to determine how your medical record system, hospital information system, and other software solutions support such identification. Again, don't forget to look toward the billing system for provider specific data. Research on the impact of NP practice in healthcare across the board focuses on Outcomes, illustrating that such data is, in fact, available (Kapu & Kleinpell, 2012).

Physician Assistants

After considering CRNAs, Midwives, and NPs, we are now ready to look at Physician Assistants, or PAs. The first PA educational programs were developed at Duke University in 1965, as a response to increasing healthcare needs in rural communities across America. Per the American Academy of Physician Assistants (AAPA), in 2010, 40% of the nearly 75,000 practicing PAs worked in hospital settings ("About AAPA," 2014).

Per CMS, a PA must be licensed by the state to practice as a PA and have either graduated from an accredited PA educational program, or have passed the national certification examination administered by the National

Commission on Certification of Physician Assistants ("Medicare information for advanced practice," 2014).

Typical hospital duties include evaluating and treating patients in the Emergency Room, performing histories and physicals, admitting patients on behalf of Physicians, providing surgical first assisting for planned and emergency operations, conducting patient rounds, evaluating changes in patients' conditions, ordering medications, treatments, and laboratory tests, and writing discharge summaries. PAs working in certain specialty areas may have additional privileges associated with the specialty ("About PA practice," 2014).

The exact requirements for physician supervision of PAs are defined by state law. All states allow for a degree of flexibility associated with off-site supervision by Physicians, provided the supervising Physician is available via telecommunication. PAs are, like their Physician supervisors and colleagues, privileged and credentialed based on the 6 general competencies prescribed by the ACGME and the American Board of Medical Specialties. The American Academy of Physician Assistants recommends that the actual privileges available to PAs be stated in the Medical Staff bylaws, rules, and regulations. Check that yours are up to date. Further, the AAPA recommends that PAs, like their supervising Physicians, be evaluated using Medical Staff processes, consistent with current accreditation standards ("About PA practice," 2014).

See Table 5.10 (p. 149) for a sample of potential core privileges for a PA. Note that these privileges may vary by state.

Once the PA's core privileges have been outlined, additional, special privileges may be added. In most situations, not all PAs will have each of these special privileges. Instead, those PAs who have achieved the appropriate training and experience may be granted those privileges that they perform in the hospital ("What is a physician," 2015). Remember that privileges should only be granted for care processes that are provided by your hospital.

Once we have the core privileges established for the PAs within the hospital, we add the special privileges as appropriate. See Table 5.11 (p. 150). Next, as we have with the previous APC groups, we develop the profiling metrics associated with this group of providers. See Table 5.12, which follows, for potential measures that may be a starting point for you.

Table 5.12 PA Profile draft

INDICATOR/MEASURE	ACGME CATEGORY	TQ DOMAIN
Complete and Timely Documentation in Medical Record (Compliance Rate)	Professionalism	Citizenship
Referrals to Supervising Physician or Specialist (Number and Percent)	Volume; Patient Care	Processes of Care
Appropriate Communication with Medical Team (Rate)	Professionalism	Citizenship
Patient Complaints (Number And Rate)	Professionalism; Patient Care	Patient Satisfaction
Patient Satisfaction; Percent Highly Satisfied or Equivalent	Professionalism; Patient Care	Patient Satisfaction
Participation in Medical Staff Committees, Projects (Percent and Rate)	Practice-Based Learning and Improvement	Citizenship
Hospital Associated Illness/ Conditions (Number and Rate)	Medical Knowledge; Patient Care	Processes of Care; Clinical Outcomes
Surgical Site Infections (Number and Rate)	Medical Knowledge; Patient Care	Processes of Care; Clinical Outcomes
Compliance with Discharge Standards (Number and Rate)	Systems-Based Practice	Volume; Processes of Care; Clinical Outcomes
Chronic Conditions Management, Identification of Additional Needs (Number and Rate)	Medical Knowledge; Acuity	Processes of Care; Volume; Clinical Outcomes
Implementation of Proper Pain/Condition Management Techniques and Monitoring (Number and Rate)	Medical Knowledge	Processes of Care
Blood/Blood Product Utilization (Rate)	Medical Knowledge	Processes of Care
Medication/Rx Utilization (Rate)	Medical Knowledge	Processes of Care
Standard, Best Practice Intervention (Rate)	Medical Knowledge; Practice-Based Learning and Improvement	Processes of Care; Privilege-Based Metrics
Patient Education Plan Compliance (Rate)	Medical; Patient Care	Processes of Care; Privilege-Based Metrics
Patient Evaluation per Standards (Compliance Rate)	Medical Knowledge; Practice-Based Learning and Improvement	Processes of Care; Privilege-Based Metrics; Volume

INDICATOR/MEASURE	ACGME CATEGORY	TQ DOMAIN
Diagnostic Testing Appropriate (Rate)	Medical Knowledge	Processes of Care; Privilege-Based Metrics
Preventative Screening Appropriate (Rate)	Medical Knowledge; Patient Care	Processes of Care; Privilege-Based Metrics
Participation in In-House Trainings; Maintenance of Certifications and Licensure (Number and Compliance Rate); CME Activity	Practice-Based Learning and Improvement; Medical Knowledge	Citizenship
Achievement of Advanced Clinical Training in Areas of Focus (Number and Percent Addressed)	Practice-Based Learning and Improvement; Medical Knowledge	Citizenship
Adjusted Cost per Case (if Attributed Provider)	Systems-Based Practice	Efficiency
Internal Satisfaction Survey Results	Interpersonal and Communication	Citizenship
Peer Reviewed Cases	Practice-Based learning and Improvement	Reviews
ALOS of Patient Population (if Attributed Provider)	Systems-Based Practice	Efficiency
Mortality Rate/Count of Patient Population (if Attributed Provider)	Patient Care	Processes of Care; Clinical Outcomes
Average CMI of Patient Population (if Attributed Provider)	Acuity	Acuity
Compliance with PA Relationship, Supervision Regulations	Systems-Based Practice; Professionalism	Citizenship
Core Measure Compliance (as Appropriate and Applicable)	Medical Knowledge	Processes of Care
Readmission Rate, Number (if Attributed Provider)	Systems-Based Practice	Efficiency; Process of Care
Noncompliance with Medical Staff Rules, Regulations	Professionalism	Citizenship; Reviews

Note that as with the previously considered APCs, attribution for PA activity may be a challenge. Your hospital may or may not attribute cases and patient care directly to PAs. There is no "one size fits all" approach to PA attribution, but it is clear upon focusing on PA profile metrics that accounting for PA activities with patients is necessary. In many cases, surveying potential data sources for billable care, bundled care, and procedural coding with appropriate attribution may result in useful data (Moote, Nelson, Vletkamp, & Campbell, 2012).

The metrics used in profiling PAs should focus on major competencies required to effectively work within their areas of practice, as TJC requires and the models provided in the preceding chapters support.

Should Physician Assistants and Nurse Practitioners Be Grouped Together?

Many patients may assume PAs and NPs are the same, as they both fall into the APC arena and seem to provide many of the same services at the hospital. In regard to the Medical Staff Office's view of these 2 groups of providers, however, differences exist.

In many states, the PA has more independence associated with her practice than her counterpart NP may have (Kess, 2011). NPs provide care based on a nursing model, while PAs are trained in what is termed a 'medical model,' which is also how Physicians are trained (Smith & Sabino, 2012). In some environments, these educational impacts may be more evident than in others; you may notice variation in your hospital's APCs. On the other hand, in some states, the opposite may be the case with NPs having more independence than PAs (Cresswell, 2014).

Despite these differences, some hospitals do in fact 'lump' PAs and NPs together, treating them as the same. In a way, this may be logical—both groups provide what may be termed an 'extension' of the reach of a physician ("Use of nonphysician clinical," 2014). For our focus in this text, what we must remember is that both NPs and PAs, as well as the other APCs considered herein, must be evaluated per OPPE standards.

Summary

In this chapter, our focus has been on Advanced Practice Clinicians (APCs). First, we examined Certified Registered Nurse Anesthetists (CRNAs), with a review of possible privilege sets and a set of 'starting point' profiling metrics. We then transitioned to an exploration of Midwife practice, focusing on Certified Nurse Midwives (CNMs) and their hospital privileges, both core and special. We proposed a starting point of profiling metrics for CNMs, realizing that for your hospital, specific variations and adjustments may be necessary.

We moved on to consider the same—core privileges, special privileges, and potential profiling metrics—for Nurse Practitioners (NPs) and Physician Assistants (PAs). We concluded this discussion on the similarities and differences associated with NPs and PAs.

Chapter 6 will explore finding data sources, and being sure that your data is Valid, Accurate, and Reliable, to create high quality profiles.

Reference List:

"About AAPA." (2014). American Academy of Physician Assistants. Retrieved from http://www.aapa.org/twocolumnmain.aspx?id=1849

"About PA practice." (2014) American Academy of Physician Assistants. Retrieved from http://www.aapa.org/twocolumnmain.aspx?id=321

"A guide to understanding state restrictions on NP practice." (2014). The Advisory Board Company. Retrieved from http://www.advisory.com/research/medical-group-strategy-council/resources/2013/understanding-state-restric-tions-on-np-practice

"All about NPs." (2014). American Association of Nurse Practitioners. Retrieved from http://www.aanp.org/all-about-nps

"Certified nurse-midwife." (2013). Medline Plus. Retrieved from http://www.nlm.nih.gov/medlineplus/ency/article/002000.htm

"Certified registered nurse anesthetist fact sheet." (2014). American Association of Nurse Anesthetists. Retrieved from http://www.aana.com/ceandeducation/beco-meacrna/Pages/Nurse-Anesthetists-at-a-Glance.aspx

Creswell, S. (2014). What's the difference between a nurse practitioner and a physician assistant and what should you choose? Gap Medics. Retrieved from http://www.gapmedics.com/blog/2013/12/23/what-s-the-difference-between-a-physician-assistant-and-a-nurse-practitioner-and-what-should-you-choose

"CRNA scope of practice." (2014). AANA. Retrieved from http://www.aana.com/aboutus/Documents/scopeofpractice.pdf

"Definition of midwifery and scope of practice of certified nurse-midwives and certified midwives." (2011). American College of Nurse-Midwives. Retrieved from http://www.midwife.org/ACNM/files/ACNMLibraryData/UPLOADFILE-NAME/000000000266/Definition%20of%20Midwifery%20and%20Scope%20of%20Practice%20of%20CNMs%20and%20CMs%20Dec%202011.pdf

"Frequently asked questions about midwives and midwifery." (2014). Citizens for Midwifery. Retrieved from http://cfmidwifery.org/midwifery/faq.aspx

"Historical timeline." (2014). American Association of Nurse Practitioners. Retrieved from http://www.aanp.org/about-aanp/historical-timeline

"History of nurse anesthesia practice." (2010). American Association of Nurse Anesthetists. Retrieved from http://www.aana.com/aboutus/documents/historynap.pdf

"Hospital practice." (2014). American Academy of Physician Assistants. Retrieved from https://www.aapa.org/threeColumnLanding.aspx?id=2172

Kapu, A.N. & Kleinpell, R. (2012). Developing nurse practitioner associated metrics for outcomes assessment. Vanderbilt University. Retrieved from http://www.mc.vanderbilt.edu/documents/CAPNAH/files/41-Developing%20np%20associated%20metrics%20for%20outcomes%20assessment.pdf

Kess, S. (2011). Nurse practitioners vs. physician assistant. *The Washington Post.* Retrieved from http://www.washingtonpost.com/wp-dyn/content/article/2011/01/07/AR2011010704936.html

Malina, D.P. & Izlar, J.J. (2014). Education and practice barriers for Certified Register Nurse Anesthetists. *The Online Journal of Issues in Nursing,* (19). Retrieved from http://www.nursingworld.org/MainMenuCategories/ANAMarketplace/ANAPeriodicals/OJIN/TableofContents/Vol-19-2014/No2-May-2014/Barriers-for-Certified-Registered-Nurse-Anesthetists.html

"Mayo School of Health Science: Nurse practitioner." (2014). Mayo Clinic. Retrieved from http://www.mayo.edu/mshs/careers/nurse-practitioner

"Medicare coverage of non-physician practitioner services." (2001). Department of Health and Human Services, Office of Inspector General. Retrieved from https://oig.hhs.gov/oei/reports/oei-02-00-00290.pdf

"Medicare information for advanced practice registered nurses, anesthesiologist assistants, and physician assistants." (2011). Medicare Learning Network, CMS. Retrieved from http://www.cms.gov/Outreach-and-Education/Medicare-Learning-Network-MLN/MLNProducts/Downloads/Medicare_Information_for_APNs_and_PAs_Booklet_ICN901623.pdf

"Midwife licensing program." (2014). Arizona Department of Health Services. Retrieved from http://azdhs.gov/als/midwife/

Moote, M., Nelson, R., Veltkamp, R., & Campbell D. (2012). Productivity assessment of physician assistants and nurse practitioners in oncology in an academic medical center. *Journal of Oncology Practice, 8* (3), 167-172. Retrieved from http://www.ncbi.nlm.nih.gov/pmc/articles/PMC3396805/

"Questions and answers—career possibilities in nurse anesthesia." (2015). American Association of Nurse Anesthetists. Retrieved from http://www.aana.com/ce-andeducation/becomeacrna/Pages/Questions-and-Answers-Career-Possibilities-in-Nurse-Anesthesia.aspx

Rhyne, J.A. (2008). Supervision of midlevel practitioners: How much is enough? *North Carolina Medical Board Forum* (3). Retrieved from http://www.ncmedboard.org/images/uploads/publications_uploads/no308.pdf

Runyon, L. (2014). The role of the Advance Practice Clinician (APC) in pediatric trauma care. Retrieved from http://www.pedtrauma.org/wp-content/uploads/2014/07/04.RUNYON-The-Role-of-the-Advance-Practice-Clinician.pdf

Sadr, A. (2014). History of midwifery. Dimensions Healthcare System. Retrieved from http://www.dimensionshealth.org/index.php/dimensions-health-services-prince-georges-county-maryland-md/midwifery/history-of-midwifery/

Schrand, S. (2014). Let Pennsylvania nurse practitioners help ease shortages. Pennslyvania Coalition of Nurse Practitioners (PACNP). Retrieved from http://www.pacnp.org/news/207650/Let-Pennsylvania-nurse-practitioners-help-ease-care-shortages.htm

Smith, D. & Sabino, T. (2012). Where's the doctor? PAs and NPs on the front lines of US healthcare. *Voices in Medical Sociology: Contemporary and Historical Perspectives*. Retrieved from http://www.academia.edu/1212332/Where_s_the_Doctor_PAs_and_NPs_on_the_Front_Lines_of_U.S._Healthcare

"Use of nonphysician clinical staff in hospitalist programs, Chapter 8." (2014). Retrieved from http://www.hospitalmedicine.org/CMDownload.aspx?ContentKey=ed0642ef-e72e-428e-bb5b-5bec8dee83d0&ContentItemKey=85c8f112-e195-4e8b-b0c0-f89f2705edf1.

"State by state." (2014). MANA: Midwives Alliance North America. Retrieved from http://mana.org/about-midwives/state-by-state

"The future of nursing: Leading change, advancing health." (2010). Institute of Medicine. Retrieved from http://www.iom.edu/reports/2010/the-future-of-nursing-leading-change-advancing-health/recommendations.aspx

"Types of midwives." (2014). AME: Association of Midwifery Educators. Retrieved from http://associationofmidwiferyeducators.org/aspiring-midwives.html

Weitz, T., Anderson, P., & Taylor, D. (2009). Advancing the scope of practice for advanced practice clinicians: More than a matter of access. Association of Reproductive Health Professionals. Retrieved from http://www.arhp.org/publications-and-resources/contraception-journal/august-2009

"What is a midwife?" (2014). MANA: Midwives Alliance North America. Retrieved from http://mana.org/about-midwives/what-is-a-midwife

"What is a physician assistant?" (2015). California Department of Consumer Affairs: Physician Assistant Board. Retrieved from http://www.pac.ca.gov/forms_pubs/what_is.shtml

NOTES

Table 5.1 Core Privileges for CRNAs draft (may vary by state)

CORE PRIVILEGE CATEGORY	PRIVILEGE
Anesthesia, Before Use	Perform and Document a Pre-Anesthetic Assessment and Evaluation of the Patient, including Requesting Consultations and Diagnostic Studies
Anesthesia, Before Use	Obtain Informed Consent for Anesthesia
Anesthesia, Before Use	Develop an Anesthesia Plan
Anesthesia, Use	Initiate the Anesthetic Technique (General, Regional, Local, Sedation)
Anesthesia, Use	Select, Apply, and Insert Appropriate Non-Invasive and Invasive Monitoring Modalities for Continuous Evaluation of the Patient's Status
Anesthesia, Use	Select, Obtain, and Administer Anesthetics, Adjuvant and Accessory Drugs, and Fluids Necessary to Manage the Anesthetic
Anesthesia, Use	Manage Patient's Airway and Pulmonary Status Using Current Practice Modalities
Anesthesia, Use	Perform Peri-Anesthetic Invasive and Non-Invasive Monitoring
Anesthesia, Recovery	Initiate and Administer Respiratory Support to Ensure Adequate Ventilation and Oxygenation in the Post-Anesthesia Period
Anesthesia, Recovery	Facilitate Emergence and Recovery from Anesthesia
Anesthesia, Recovery	Discharge the Patient from Post-Anesthesia Care Area, and Provide Post-Anesthesia Follow Up Evaluation and Care
Emergency Response	Respond to Emergency Situations by Providing Airway Management, Administration of Emergency Fluids and Drugs, and Use of Basic or Advanced Cardiac Life Support Techniques
Appropriate Patient Care	Manage Peripheral Intravenous Catheters
Appropriate Patient Care	Manage Mechanical Ventilation/Oxygen Therapy
Appropriate Patient Care	Recognize Abnormal Patient Response During Anesthesia, Selecting and Implementing Corrective Actions
Appropriate Patient Care	Initiate and Administer Pharmacological or Fluid Support of the Cardiovascular System
Pain Management	Order, Initiate, or Modify Pain Relief Therapy, through the Utilization of Drugs, Regional Anesthesia, or Other Accepted Modalities
Appropriate Patient Care	Insert Intravenous Lines
Appropriate Patient Care	Insert and Manage Arterial Lines and Perform Arterial Puncture to Obtain Arterial Blood Samples

CORE PRIVILEGE CATEGORY	PRIVILEGE
Appropriate Patient Care	Insert and Manage Pulmonary Artery Catheters, Peripheral and Central IV Catheters
Anesthesia, Use	Obtain, Prepare, and Use All Equipment, Monitors, Supplies, and Drugs Used for the Administration of Anesthesia and Sedation, Performing and Ordering Safety Checks as Needed
Emergency Response	Perform CPR
Airway Management	Perform Tracheal Intubation, including Laryngoscopy, Fiberoptic Bronchoscopy, Laryngeal Mask Airway Assisted Intubation, and Crichothyrotomy
Pain Management	Place Epidural Blood Patch for Post-Dural Puncture Headache
Appropriate Patient Care	Administer Blood Products after Obtaining a Hematocrit and Consulting with Anesthesiologist
Emergency Response	Perform Emergency Endotracheal Intubations
Appropriate Patient Care	Obtain Informed Consent for Blood, Blood Products, and Procedures Institutionally Privileged to Perform

Table 5.2 Special Privileges for CRNAs draft

SPECIAL PRIVILEGE CATEGORY	PRIVILEGE
Anesthesia Use	Diagnostic and Therapeutic Injections with or without Fluoroscopic Guidance, including Epidural, Caudal, Spinal, Facet Joint, Selective Nerve, and Sympathetic Blocks
Appropriate Patient Care	Limited Ultrasound for Guided Procedure
Anesthesia Use	Pediatric Sedation
Pain Management	Acute and Chronic Pain Therapy
Emergency Response, Appropriate Patient Care	Participate in Advanced Cardiac Life Support Efforts, While Maintaining Current ACLS Certification
Appropriate Patient Care	Insertion/Removal of Peripheral Arterial Catheters
Anesthesia Use	Intravenous Regional Anesthesia Block Management
Anesthesia Use	Lumbar Epidural Anesthesia/Analgesia Management
Anesthesia Use	Subarachnoid Block Anesthesia Management

Table 5.4 Core Privileges for CNMs draft (may vary by state)

CORE PRIVILEGE CATEGORY	PRIVILEGE
Birth Management	Perform Artificial Rupture of Membranes
Birth Management	Apply: External Scalp Monitor, Fetal Scalp Electrode, Intrauterine Pressure Catheter as Indicated
Birth Management	Perform Normal Spontaneous Vaginal Delivery with or without an Episiotomy
Birth Management	Order/Monitor Oxytocin for Augmentation or Induction After Consultation
Birth Management	Order Administration of Vitamin K 1mg IM Before 1 Hour of Age
Birth Management	Administer Prostaglandin Gel for Cervical Ripening
Birth Management; Infant Care	Monitor Mother and Infant Vital Signs as Appropriate
General Patient Care	Perform Hospital Admissions, Rounds, Discharges
Birth Management; General Patient Care	Alert Consulting/Supervising Physician of Emergent and/or Non-Emergent Needs
Birth Management; General Patient Care	Collaborate with Healthcare Team; Consult with OB or GYN (or Other Physician/Specialist) as Appropriate
General Patient Care	Provide Family Planning Information and Services to Patients and Families
General Patient Care	Diagnose, Evaluate, and Treat Basic Vaginal Infections, Not Associated with Medical Complications or Sexually Transmitted Diseases and/or Threatening Behaviors
General Patient Care	Screen Patients for Sexual Abuse, and Domestic Violence, per Hospital Policy
General Patient Care	Educate Patients and Families on Sexually Transmitted Diseases and High-Risk Behaviors
General Patient Care	Perform Basic Gynecological and Pelvic Exams
General Patient Care	Provide Information to Parents of Maturing Adolescent/Pre-Adolescent Females on Hormones, Maturation, Menstruation, and Development
General Patient Care	Prescribe Birth Control Medications, Treatments, and Interventions
General Patient Care	Prescribe Appropriate Medications for Treatment of Gynecological or Menopausal Concerns/Needs
General Patient Care	Perform Pap Smear and Cultures, Clinical Pelvimetry, Fern Testing, Fetal Fibronectin
Birth Management	Administer Local Block for Delivery
Birth Management	Order IV Therapy to Maintain Hydration of Patient
Infant Care	Clamp and Cut the Umbilical Cord; Obtain Specimen of Cord Blood
General Patient Care	Diagnose and Treat Vaginitis and UTIs

CORE PRIVILEGE CATEGORY	PRIVILEGE
General Patient Care	Sign the Birth Certificate
Professional Commitment	Document All Activities, Procedures, Interventions, and Patient Care Provisions per Hospital Policy

Table 5.6 Special Privileges for CNMs draft

SPECIAL PRIVILEGE CATEGORY	PRIVILEGE
Post-Birth Patient Care	Repair of Third, Fourth Degree Lacerations
General Patient Care	Perform Colonoscopy
General Patient Care	Perform Hysterosalpingogram
Post-Birth Patient Care	Manually Remove Placenta
Birth Management	Apply Vacuum Extractor in the Presence of Attending Physician
Specialized Patient Care	Perform Endometrial Biopsy
Specialized Patient Care	Perform Cervical and Endocervical Biopsy and Cryotherapy
Specialized Patient Care	Insert and Remove Subcutaneous Progestin Implants
Birth Management	Initially Manage Patients with Preeclampsia or Premature Onset of Labor (<35 Weeks)
Post-Birth Patient Care	Order/Perform Oxytocin Challenge Test
Birth Management	Administer Epidural Anesthesia
Specialized Patient Care	Perform Amnioinfusion
General Patient Care	Perform Basic Ultrasound Examinations
Infant Care	Circumcise Newborns
Post-Birth Patient Care	Manage Fetal Demise
Birth Management	Act as 1st Assist with C-Section
Generalized Patient Care; Specialized Patient Care	Act as 1st Assist with Other Surgeries Associated With Population and Scope of Care
Birth Management	Administer Pitocin for Induction or Augmentation of Labor
General Patient Care; Specialized Patient Care	Collaborate with Endocrinology/Diabetes Care for Gestational Diabetes Patients
General Patient Care; Specialized Patient Care	Collaboratively Manage Multiple-Fetus Pregnancies
General Patient Care; Specialized Patient Care	Term Labor with Fetal Abnormality
Specialized Patient Care	Collaboratively Plan/Manage/Monitor Fertility Treatments
Specialized Patient Care	Monitor/Manage Maternal Airway and Vital Signs During Labor

145

Table 5.7 Core Privileges for NPs draft (may vary by state)

CORE PRIVILEGE CATEGORY	PRIVILEGE
General Patient Care	Obtain a Relevant Health, Medical, and Psych History
General Patient Care	Perform a Physical Examination
General Patient Care	Conduct Preventative Screenings; Identify Medical and Health Risks/Needs
Documentation/Professionalism	Update/Record Changes in Health Status; Document All Clinical Findings and Records of Care
General Patient Care	Formulate the Appropriate Differential Diagnosis Based on History, Physical Examination, and Clinical Findings
General Patient Care	Identify Needs of Individual, Family, or Community as a Result of Evaluation of Collected Data
General Patient Care	Order and Interpret/Act upon Appropriate Diagnostic Tests
General Patient Care	Identify Appropriate Pharmacological Agents; Identify Non-Pharmacological Interventions
General Patient Care	Develop a Patient Education Plan
General Patient Care	Assess All Patients in Order to Determine If More Definitive Services Are Necessary
General Patient Care	Prescribe Pharmacological Agents (If NP Has Prescribing Ability)
General Patient Care	Consult with Physician and Other Healthcare Providers
General Patient Care	Determine Effectiveness of Plan of Care through Documentation of Patient Care Outcomes
Quality Improvement	Participate in Quality Assurance Review on a Periodic Basis
Documentation/Professionalism	Write Appropriate Pre- and Post-Operative Orders
General Patient Care; Emergency Response	Assess, Stabilize, and Determine the Disposition of Patients with Emergent Conditions/Needs
General Patient Care	Monitor and Manage Stable Acute and Chronic Illnesses of Patient Population
General Patient Care; Specialized Patient Care	Provide Blood Glucose Point of Care Testing, Hemoglobin A1C Point of Care Testing, Influenza Point of Care Testing, Mononucleosis Point of Care Testing
General Patient Care; Specialized Patient Care	Provide Pregnancy, PSV, Strep A, Urinalysis, Fecal Occult Blood, and Pertussis Point of Care Testing
General Patient Care; Specialized Patient Care	Evaluate, Treat, and Manage Appropriate Follow Up for Patients with Upper Respiratory Problems, UTIs, Rashes, Minor Head Injuries, Minor Blunt Trauma, and Simple Lacerations
Specialized Patient Care	Manage/Place Central Line
General Patient Care	Discharge Patients with Discharge Plans
Specialized Patient Care	Insert and Remove Foley Catheter

CORE PRIVILEGE CATEGORY	PRIVILEGE
General Patient Care	Insert and Remove IVs
General Patient Care	Perform Minor Surgical Procedures Such as Punch Biopsy, Sebaceous Cyst and Ingrown Toenail Removal, and Repair of Minor Lacerations
General Patient Care	Manage Non-Displaced Fractures and Sprains, Including Casting and Insertion/Removal of Drains
General Patient Care	Assist Sponsoring/Supervising Physician in Surgery or With Other Treatment Procedures
Specialized Patient Care	Care for Indwelling Vascular Catheters, Chest Tubes, Gastrostomy Tubes, Gastrojejunostomy Tubes, Cecostomy Tubes, Sclerotherapy Tubes, and Abscess Drainage Tubes
General Patient Care	Initiate Requests for Commonly Performed Laboratory Studies
General Patient Care; Specialized Patient Care	Assess and Manage Common Chronic Conditions (Such as Diabetes Mellitus or High Blood Pressure) as Indicated by Supervising Physician
General Patient Care	Provide Immunizations as Appropriate
General Patient Care	Providing Screening Tests as Appropriate; Interpret Results and Counsel Patient/Family

Table 5.8 Special Privileges for NPs draft

SPECIAL PRIVILEGE CATEGORY	PRIVILEGE
Specialized Patient Care	Place PICCs
Specialized Patient Care	Perform Colonoscopies
Specialized Patient Care	Perform Endometrial Biopsies
Specialized Patient Care	Perform Umbilical Artery/Venous Catheterization
General Patient Care	Initiate and Manage Intubation
Specialized Patient Care	Place and Remove Chest Tubes
Specialized Patient Care	Perform Lumbar Punctures
Specialized Patient Care	Monitor and Manage Chest Pain
Specialized Patient Care; General Patient Care	Perform Pharmacological/Non-Pharmacological Stress Tests
Specialized Patient Care; General Patient Care	Assist in Surgery to include First Assist, Deep and Simplified Tissue Closures, Application of Appliances, and Other Actions Dictated by Surgeon
Specialized Patient Care	Harvest Sapheneous Vein or Radial Artery Conduit
Specialized Patient Care	Insert Radial and Femoral Arterial Lines
Specialized Patient Care	Insert Intra-Aortic Balloon Pump
Specialized Patient Care	Change G-Tubes
Specialized Patient Care	Manage Epistaxis
Specialized Patient Care	Initiate/Manage Cardioversion
Specialized Patient Care	Remove Temporary Pacemaker Wires
Specialized Patient Care	Remove Intra-Aortic Balloon Pump
Patient Care Preparation	Prepare Implantation Tissue
Patient Care Preparation	Prepare Autologous Grafts
Specialized Patient Care	Administer Intrathecal Chemotherapy
Specialized Patient Care	Perform/Interpret Nuclear Medicine Shutogram Studies
Specialized Patient Care	Provide Needle Thoracotomy
Specialized Patient Care	Diagnose and Manage Treatment of Complicated Complications or Comorbidities

Table 5.10 Core Privileges for PAs draft (may vary by state)

CORE PRIVILEGE CATEGORY	PRIVILEGE
General Patient Care	Perform Initial and Ongoing Assessment of Patients' Medical, Physical, and Psychiatric Status
General Patient Care	Perform and Document Complete Physical Examination
General Patient Care	Record Diagnostic Impressions; Treat Based on Applicable Standards
General Patient Care	Write Orders for Diagnostic Tests, Activities, Therapies, Diet, and Vital Signs, Drugs, IV Fluids, Blood and Blood Products, Oxygen, and Consultations
General Patient Care	Instruct, Educate, and Counsel Patients on Health Status, Results of Tests, Disease Process, Discharge Summaries, and Planning
General Patient Care	Evaluate Interim Patient Status and Document in the Progress Notes
General Patient Care	Initiate Consultation by Other Physicians at the Direction of the Supervising Physician
General Patient Care; Specialized Patient Care	Implement Physician Directed Treatment Plans, as Applicable
General Patient Care; Specialized Patient Care	Recognize and Evaluate Situations Requiring Immediate Attention and Institute, when Necessary, Treatment Procedures Essential for the Life of the Patient, including BCLS; Notify Supervising Physician Immediately
General Patient Care	Apply Splints and Casts
General Patient Care	Suture Minor Lacerations
General Patient Care	Deliver Care Under Pre-Approved Protocols That Have Been Reviewed and Accepted by the Supervising Physician and Appropriate Medical Staff Committees
General Patient Care; Specialized Patient Care	Prescribe/Dispense Pharmacological Interventions (if Prescribing is Authorized)
General Patient Care	Immunize Patients per Protocol
General Patient Care	Screen Patients Based on Identified Needs, Challenges, Environment, and Presenting Issues
General Patient Care	Monitor Vital Signs and Related Predictors of Status
General Patient Care	Admit, Round, and Discharge Patients (if Applicable/ Authorized)
General Patient Care	Develop a Patient Care Plan; Implement and Monitor
General Patient Care; Specialized Patient Care	Develop a Discharge Plan; Coordinate with Appropriate Parties

Table 5.11 Special Privileges for PAs draft

SPECIAL PRIVILEGE CATEGORY	PRIVILEGE
Specialized Patient Care	Insert/Remove/Monitor Chest Tubes, G-Tubes
Specialized Patient Care	Insert Central Lines; Monitor
Specialized Patient Care	Perform Endotracheal Intubation; Monitor; Remove
General Patient Care	Perform Fractural Splinting
Specialized Patient Care	Provide Anesthesia (Class 1), including Local Infiltration and Topical Application, Minor Nerve Blocks; Administer Sedative and Analgesic Drugs
Specialized Patient Care	Assist in Labor and Delivery
Specialized Patient Care	Assist in the Management of Injuries, Emergent and Chronic Conditions
Specialized Patient Care	Perform Spinal Tab/Lumbar Puncture
Specialized Patient Care	Perform Paracentesis, Thoracentesis
Specialized Patient Care	Aspirate Bone Marrow; Perform Biopsy
General Patient Care	Perform Well-Woman Exams and Pap Smear
Specialized Patient Care	Establish, Maintain/Monitor, and Remove Percutaneous Venous and Arterial Lines
Specialized Patient Care	Perform Arterial Cutdowns
Specialized Patient Care	Insert Balloon Pump
Specialized Patient Care	Perform Open Vein Harvesting
Specialized Patient Care	Remove Pacemaker Wires
Specialized Patient Care	Manage/Perform Endoscopic Vein Harvesting
Specialized Patient Care	Order/Interpret Atypical Patient Tests, Including PET Scans, Pharmacological/Non-Pharmacological Stress Tests, and Octreotide Scans
Specialized Patient Care	Collaboratively Evaluate Patients in the Organ Donation/Transplant Process

NOTES

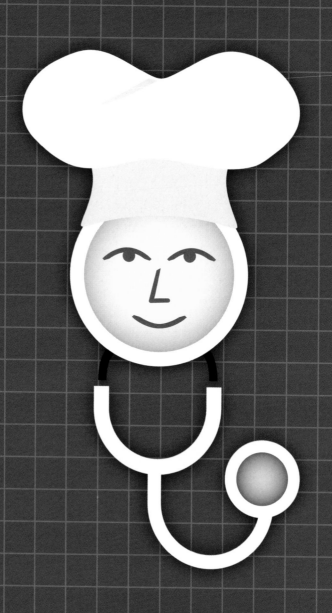

Chapter 6
Shopping for Ingredients: Seeking Quality Data

Let's Go Shopping!

Now that we know our diners, and have at least a preliminary menu planned, it's time to go shopping for the ingredients we need. Chances are we have already looked for what is available (the search for data sources with the correct data fields) to be sure we can prepare what is on our menu.

When it comes to shopping for our data, we can be assured that most of our ingredients will be available in a large grocery store or outlet (think large discharge database here). Others, however, will require trips around town to smaller "boutique" stores with specialized ingredients (think Pathology and Radiology here). Start with the big grocery, grab a cart, and let's go up and down the aisles!

We need to be sure that our ingredients are just what we need – garlic won't work if our recipe calls for onions – and we need to check the quality of our items. Thump those melons; check every can for its expiration date.

Just like a fine restaurant, you want the local Department of Health hanging an A rating on your wall. You may have designed the best menu around, but if the milk is sour or the eggs go bad, you will lose your customers fast!

Finally, remember that we will need to push our basket through the checkout line, paying for everything. Be careful that your selections match your budget – there may be some items that you cannot afford (think complex measures that are resource intensive or require lengthy patient follow up). This experience may be frustrating, but in the long-run, your customers will understand.

Remember that it is okay to start small. It is better to offer a small meal that is really good than to get bogged down with a kitchen full of ingredients that end up in a stew that your diners will ignore or review badly online.

Now that we have a pretty good idea of who we are profiling, and what will be included on the profiles, our next task is to build them. We need to start with the data itself.

▉ Data Sources

For most providers in the inpatient setting who take on the role of Admitting, Attending, Consulting, or Procedure Provider (principal or secondary procedures), the best single source for data is the file created after the patient is discharged. This data is based on the abstracted and coded medical record. Often knows as "administrative data," this dataset is in a uniform format used for billing. The current version, UB-04, has been approved by the National Uniform Billing Committee (NUBC).

The NUBC was formed by the American Hospital Association in 1975, after almost 10 years of failed attempts to create a standardized billing form in the United States. The NUBC, comprised of a broad coalition of industry members, including the Health Care Financing Administration, now known as the Center for Medicare and Medicaid Services (CMS), continued this work. In 1982, it accepted the first national standardized billing dataset, designated UB-82. After an 8-year moratorium on changes, the dataset was updated with design improvements in 1992, and designated UB-92. Further enhancements were approved in 2004, creating our current standard, UB-04 ("About the NUBC," 2014).

UB-04, used by institutional providers, includes all the elements identified as necessary for claims processing. In addition, it functions as the source for new data fields for electronic billing formats. Compared to UB-92, UB-04 includes the following enhancements:

- Expansion of fields to accommodate ICD-10-CM codes, both for diagnoses and procedures
- Fields to designate if a diagnosis was present on admission (POA) or Not Present on Admission (NPOA), a data element mandated by the Deficit Reduction Act of 2005, and required for inpatient prospective payment system hospitals since October 2007; the NPOA flag designates those diagnoses that occurred after admission, perhaps indicating a complication of therapy
- Expansion of the number of fields for diagnoses from 9 to 18, improving the value of the data for reporting and analysis of patient populations
- Revised physician fields, including a distinct field for the National Provider Identifier (NPI)

Although UB-04 is standardized, individual states, government agencies, and insurers create their own versions, as a quick "UB-04 tour" of the Internet demonstrates. The following is a high level summary of the types of data in UB-04 that we have identified as relevant for provider profiling, roughly in ascending order of the field numbers:

- Billing provider information
- Patient information, including medical record number, address, date of birth, and gender
- Admission date and time, type of admission, and source
- Discharge date and hour
- Discharge status (home, rehabilitation, skilled nursing, deceased, etc.)
- Total charges
- Provider identifiers
- Insurance information
- ICD version indicator (for example, ICD-9 or ICD-10, with the version)
- Principal diagnosis code and POA indicator (principal diagnosis, by definition, is always present on admission)
- Secondary diagnoses with POA indicators
- Admitting diagnosis (once again, this is always POA)
- External cause of injury code(s), with POA indicator(s)
- Principal procedure
- Other procedures (up to 5)
- Attending Physician
- Surgeons
- Other providers ("Key points," 2014).

Given that this information is uniformly collected and maintained, the first place to look for provider data is your own internal coding and billing systems; these are, after all, the repositories of the UB-04's data, often in a more user-friendly format. Further, these may be integrated into an electronic medical record within your hospital or organization, yielding additional benefits of related data being maintained consistently. It is important to note that your hospital's internal data set may include more fields than those defined by UB-04. For example, your system may list all procedures, not just the top 6, with provider attribution for each. In this situation, your software's inclusions are beneficial to consider when making decisions about what may be used for provider profiling based on the software's unique functional capabilities.

After delving into the data available in coding and billing systems within your hospital, you may move on to the hospital's financial cost accounting system(s). Some hospitals use software that captures all charge items associated with a care encounter; these typically exist for the facility's inpatient encounters, though outpatient may be included as well. Typically, charge data includes the individual items that would end up on a detailed bill, such as drugs given, room charges, and time billed in the Operating Room. A cost accounting system creates a cost associated with each item, in addition to the listed price. Different systems use different methodologies, but in general they attribute direct and indirect costs, including building costs, labor, and materials to each item. This data can be useful to estimate costs associated with an admission or procedure, and, with good provider attribution, can be used to compare Utilization of Services by providers. These calculations can be especially helpful when looking at the total cost of a defined procedure, such as Total Knee Replacement, and variations in cost by Surgeon. As bundled payment arrangements become more popular, these types of analyses become more important. At the same time, as more traditional revenue cycle management shifts to focus on 'true margins' and actual cost of care, advanced cost accounting is more and more necessary (Michelson, 2014). With the goal of being able to account for procedure-level costs, hospitals also take into account variation of service mix and outcomes (Azoulay et. al, 2007). Check with your hospital's finance department to see if your hospital uses a cost accounting system. If it does, explore its data to determine how best to use it in profiles.

Another good source of provider data is the billing dataset the providers use. These systems commonly use Current Procedure Terminology (CPT) codes (© 2015 American Medical Association. All rights reserved). This code set, maintained and distributed by the AMA, describes medical procedures and services, often at a very granular level. For example, whereas ICD-9 procedure codes may broadly define an Upper Gastrointestinal Endoscopy, the CPT system defines it by portions of the stomach and intestine examined, and whether specific interventions like Biopsy or Polypectomy were performed[1].

In addition to the specificity provided by the coding, billing data sets tend to be comprehensive and complete, capturing activity over a broad range of services and locations ("Code sets," 2014). Of note is that changes occur in the code set annually; remaining up to date is vital for most optimal use and acceptability (Torrey, 2015).

The next place to look for data is information systems dedicated to support Processes of Care, including care management, case management, quality, risk, and safety. These software solutions generally accept data feeds from administrative and cost accounting systems, amassing related data in one place, making it easier to build measures for provider profiling from a single dataset. In addition, these systems often support the day-to-day work of quality and case managers, allowing the entry of data on safety and risk events, infection control issues, and ad hoc data entry for quality improvement projects. Events that warrant Peer Review may also be tracked here, with the results entered; this important, provider-attributed data is then available for reporting at the discretion of the Medical Staff. With the proper data feeds and interfaces, a well-functioning system that works within this arena can be the major source of data for provider profiles. Further, these systems often support reporting of Core Measures for TJC and/or CMS requirements, providing additional metrics on best practice, by provider. The data harvest required for national reporting often includes a blinded version of the UB-04 data for all discharges, allowing the vendor to offer comparative data for benchmarking, a valuable feature when building profiles.

Some hospitals use Enterprise Resource Planning solutions, termed ERPs, that store data which can be used in provider profiles. ERPs have not, however, been fully integrated into the healthcare arena (Sanja, 2013); if your hospital has an ERP, we suggest you explore its data offerings.

Although the large administrative datasets described above are probably your best source of data for the Generic Profile outlined in Chapter 2, as a whole, they won't help you much with Pathology, Radiology, Emergency Medicine, and Anesthesiology; billing data sets may be the possible exception to this statement. In addition, it is likely that administrative data alone will

---

[1]For more information on the CPT-4 codes, please contact the American Medical Association (AMA), http://www.ama-assn.org/ama

not provide the depth of clinical information needed for robust measurement of specialty privileges, such as Gastrointestinal Endoscopy, Interventional Cardiology, or Cardiac Surgery. For these specialties, look for "boutique" datasets, which broadly fall into 2 categories.

The first of these includes the transactional systems that reside in specialty labs or the Operating Rooms. For example, Video Endoscopy Systems usually include hardware and software that not only record selected portions of the procedure, but also support the entry of patient information, and the automatic creation of procedure reports. These systems have databases that can be of further benefit, as they may support the reporting of procedure Volume by provider. Additional process metrics, such as the Duration of the Procedure and Interventions Performed, may also be available. Do an inventory of your hospital's systems, with the help of your IT team, to determine where these systems reside and if there is data available that you may wish to include in the specialty profiles. Always remember that provider profiling is by and for the Medical Staff, so work closely with your specialties as you identify and explore these datasets.

The second area to explore consists of specialty focused cooperative databases in which your hospital and Medical Staff may participate. One of the first databases was the Society of Thoracic Surgeons (STS) National Database; it was established in 1989 as an initiative for quality improvement and patient safety among Cardiothoracic Surgeons. Its national database now includes 3 components, Adult Cardiac, General Thoracic, and Congenital Heart Surgery ("STS National Database," 2014).

The American Medical Association sponsors the National Quality Registry Network (NQRN), a voluntary network of organizations operating registries and others interested in increasing the usefulness of clinical registries to measure and improve patient health outcomes. The AMA maintains a list of all active registries. A review of current registries indicates that certain professional organizations are taking the lead, sponsoring several registries ("About NQRN," 2014). Clinical registries that may be helpful for provider profiling include many on the list that follows. We recommend that you explore the entire list, which is maintained by the AMA (©2015 American Medical Association. All Rights Reserved) ("National Clinical Registry," 2014).

- American College of Cardiology:
    - o Action Registry – Get With The Guidelines (GWTG): procedure and condition registry for patients with the 2 major types of heart attacks, STEMI and NSTEMI
    - o Carotid Artery Revascularization and Endarterectomy (CARE) Registry: Procedure and condition registry for Carotid Artery Stenting and Endarterectomy procedures
    - o CathPCI Registry (Percutaneous Coronary Intervention Registry): Procedure and condition registry for diagnostic catheterization and PCI procedures
    - o Impact Registry: Procedure, condition, and disease registry for Congenital Heart Disease treated with Diagnostic Catheterizations and Catheter-based interventions
    - o Pinnacle Registry: Procedure and condition registry for Cardiology
- American College of Chest Physicians:
    - o Bronchoscopy Diagnostic Registry: Procedure registry for Diagnostic Bronchoscopy procedures
    - o Bronchoscopy Interventional Registry: Procedure registry for Interventional Bronchoscopy procedures
- American College of Radiology:
    - o National Radiology Data Registry/CT Colonography Registry (CTC): Procedure registry for CT Colonography procedures
    - o National Radiology Data Registry/Dose Index Registry: Procedure registry for reporting CT Dose Index
    - o National Radiology Data Registry/General Radiology Improvement Database (GRID): Procedure registry for Radiology procedures
    - o National Radiology Data Registry/National Mammography Database (NMD): Procedure registry for Mammography procedures
- American College of Surgeons:
    - o Metabolic Bariatric Surgery Accreditation Quality Improvement Program Registry: Procedure registry for Bariatric Surgery procedures
    - o National Surgical Quality Improvement Project Registry (NSQIP): Procedure registry for Surgery
    - o National Trauma Registry: Health services registry for Trauma
    - o Surgeon Specific Registry: Procedure registry for Surgical procedures

- American Gastroenterological Association:
    - o Colorectal Cancer Screening and Surveillance Registry: Procedure registry for Gastroenterology
    - o Digestive Health Outcomes Registry: Procedure and condition registry for Gastroenterology
- American Society of Plastic Surgeons:
    - o Tracking Operations and Outcomes for Plastic Surgeons (TOPS) Registry: Procedure registry for Plastic Surgery
- American Society of Anesthesiologists/Anesthesia Quality Institute:
    - o Anesthesia Awareness Registry: Condition and procedure registry for Anesthesia
    - o National Anesthesia Clinical Outcomes Registry: Procedure registry for Anesthesiology
- Society for Vascular Surgery:
    - o Vascular Quality Initiative: Procedure registry for Vascular Surgery
- Society of Thoracic Surgery (STS):
    - o STS National Database: Procedure registry for Cardiothoracic Surgery
- Society of Transplant Surgeons:
    - o Scientific Registry of Transplant Recipients: Procedure registry for Solid Organ Transplantation
- American Heart Association:
    - o GWTG Resuscitation Registry: Health services registry for Resuscitation
    - o GWTG Stroke Registry: Condition registry for Stroke
- Kaiser Permanente:
    - o Spine Registry: Device registry for Spinal Implants
    - o Hip Fracture Registry: Condition registry for Hip Fractures
    - o Total Joint Replacement Registry: Procedure/device registry for Hip and Knee Replacement procedures, and device surveillance for Hip and Knee Replacements
    - o Heart Valve Registry: Procedure registry for Heart Valve surgical procedures

The above is a not a full list of registries that could be beneficial for your profiling practice. However, we are providing it as a starting point of registries that are comprehensive within a specialty and therefore potentially useful as a source of data on provider performance by privilege.

Validity, Accuracy and Reliability

At this point, we have identified an array of potential sources of data; these include the administrative UB-04 data stream, cost accounting systems, provider billing systems, quality management systems, niche clinical systems within the hospital, and cooperative databases run by professional organizations. Now, it's time to move on to the next step, which is to ensure that the data is what you were aiming to access, and that it will allow you to create measures that are Valid, Accurate, and Reliable.

Validity:

A measure is Valid if it measures what it is supposed to measure. For example, if you want to measure how often the post-operative course of an elective procedure does not go as intended, you may want to track the Number of Returns to the Operating Room During the Same Admission. Is this a Valid measure of post-operative care? The answer to this question is not as clear-cut as it may seem; in reality, the answer is "it depends." Factors that may alter the Validity of this measure include:

- Emergency cases, such as complicated trauma, that require multiple operative interventions during one admission; regardless of the quality of the care, these patients will return to the OR
- A second procedure that is elective, but happens to occur during the same admission as the principal procedure

To avoid these problems, we may want to measure the Returns to the OR only in a population of elective procedures, avoiding Emergencies and Trauma (restrictions on cases that qualify for the denominator). At the same time, we likely want to avoid elective second cases (restrictions on cases that quality for the numerator).

In terms of Validity, we may initially assess if a measure 'on its face' looks to measure what we intend; this is a measure of Face Validity (Trochim, 2006). Once we have built a measure that satisfies Face Validity, we must compare and contrast the indicator against a real data stream, checking the results. Basically, we need to verify that the Returns to the OR indicate a potential care issue. This process includes checking that the denominator – all qualifying cases – is correct, and does not unintentionally include minor surgery cases done in the Emergency Room. We also must check that the numerator, the Returns to the OR, are in fact returns on that same admission and not an occasional minor surgery procedure done on a patient transferred to rehabilitation.

Validity:

Validity expresses the degree to which a measurement measures what it purports to measure. There is extensive literature on validity in measurement, much of it by research discipline (for example, for experimental psychology). The single discipline that may be the most helpful for health-related data is Clinical Epidemiology; the following is offered as a guide, from *A Dictionary of Epidemiology, Fourth Edition*, edited by John M. Last (2001, 184, 68):

- Construct Validity: The extent to which the measurement corresponds to theoretical concepts or constructs concerning the phenomenon under study. For example, if based on theoretical grounds, the measure should change with age; thus, a measurement with Construct Validity should reflect a change with age.
- Content Validity: The extent to which the measurement incorporates the domain of the phenomenon under study. For example, a measurement of functional health status should embrace activities of daily living (occupational, family, and social functioning, etc.).
- Criterion Validity: The extent to which the measurement correlates with an external criterion of the phenomenon under study.
- Face Validity: The extent to which a measurement appears reasonable on superficial inspection, on "the face of it."

Although Face Validity is, by definition, the most superficial of these forms, it is important when seeking consensus among providers on profile measures. The measure should make sense.

Accuracy:

Accuracy is the degree to which a measurement represents the true value. Some classic examples of Accuracy are measurements of blood pressure, temperature, and tire pressure. Note that these all involve the use of gauges or sensors. The value the gauge reports can be checked against a standard to be sure the measurement is Accurate. A more relevant example for provider profiling is the common metric of Number of Inpatients Cared for by Provider per Year. One of the most common ways to get this Count is from the UB-04 administrative dataset, based on the Attending Provider field. However, the Accuracy of this measure is dependent on how the Attending Provider is determined, and if this determination is then properly coded within the dataset. Thus, the Accuracy of this data may depend on the Medical Staff policy that determines who the Attending Provider is, the chart abstraction and coding in the Health Information System, the way this data is entered into the hospital's IT system, its storage, its transfer to other systems, and, finally, how it is reported within the provider profile (Last, 2001).

A Word about Precision:

A term commonly confused with accuracy is Precision. A measure is Accurate if it states the true value, without detail. A temperature of 37.5 degrees Centigrade may be Accurate, but a more Precise value would be 37.543 degrees Centigrade. Precision is important when differences in detail matter. For the kind of data and level of detail required for provider profiling, issues of Precision rarely arise.

Reliability:

A measure is said to be Reliable when it is stable; that is, when repeated, the measure yields the same result, the measure may be thus described. High Reliability is very important for measures used for physician profiling for a major reason many who work with providers will recognize: the data has the potential to influence a provider's privileges—his or her ability to care for patients. Therefore, providers demand that they are judged by Reliable data. This is not an untenable expectation, though ensuring Reliable data is not as easy as one may hope. Potential issues in Reliability may occur when a combination of subjective and objective criteria are used to determine an attribute of an admission, for example, in the abstraction and coding of a medical record; although medical coding professionals are highly trained and conscientious, coding is nevertheless being done by human beings. It may, therefore, be subject to variation. In addition, coding conventions may change over time, impacting coding results. Also, coding is dependent on algorithms based in software systems; these may change for a range of reasons, including software updates and bug fixes.

All 3 qualities - Validity, Accuracy, and Reliability - should be part of an ongoing performance improvement initiative in your hospital. This ongoing initiative should be inclusive of departments that use and produce data, including Medical Records and Coding, Quality Assurance, Risk Management, the Medical Staff Office, and Information Technology, to name a few. The team should keep track of all the data sources being used for provider profiles, and actively monitor the coding, data entry, storage, transmission, and reporting processes to avoid problems in advance, and quickly identify and rectify them when they occur. Challenges associated with data used for reporting can seriously undermine all the best efforts to build trust in the profiles among your providers. For more on how to build your team, see Chapter 7.

Risk Adjustment

The nature of clinical medicine is that each person is a complex mixture of genetics and environment, making each individual slightly different from the next. Although we celebrate these differences every day, when it comes time to measure how providers perform for the relief of suffering and restoration of health, these differences make the task of objective, fair comparison of Outcomes difficult.

Adjustment of Risk related to Outcomes has been a major task for healthcare researchers, where the Outcomes of interest may be influenced by multiple factors. Some of these may act as confounding variables, with many known, but some unknown. One approach guaranteed to minimize confounding variation is the randomized controlled trial, wherein the intervention can be studied in 2 populations randomly selected, assuring the chance that a patient has any given variable will occur randomly. However, the population of patients who present to your hospital is anything but random, and it is common for providers, as well as hospitals, to proclaim loudly, "my/our patients are sicker!"

The single biggest effort to adjust for Resource Consumption (Days in Hospital and Resources Used) has been to create clinically coherent groups of patients based on diagnoses that appear to use the same level of resources. The original work on this was led by Fetter and Thompson at Yale University in the 1970s, and led to the original collection of Diagnosis Related Groups (DRGs), adopted by Medicare for reimbursement in the early 1980s. The CMS DRGs have gone through several iterations, with MS-DRGs being the current grouping methodology. The DRGs are clinically coherent groups, such as Myocardial Infarction, Pneumonia, or Hip Replacement, which are considered to consume the same level of resources within each group. Each DRG is assigned a Relative Weight (RW), which, when multiplied by a dollar amount unique for each hospital, determines reimbursement from CMS. DRG categories with higher weights are considered to have patients with greater Severity of Illness who, in turn, require more resources. Although useful for billing by CMS, the MS-DRGs are limited in that they are focused predominantly on patients covered by Medicare, generally 65 years old or older, and make no attempt to predict Mortality.

The original version of DRGs was extended to all patients, including children, for state Medicaid programs, becoming the All Patient, or AP-DRGs, in the late 1980s. APR-DRGs, All Patient Refined Diagnostic Related Groups, were developed next, employing clinically coherent groups with 4 levels for Severity of Illness, and 4 levels for Risk of Mortality. APR-DRGs are a product of the 3M Company, with the methodology recently expanded to create adjustment categories for Complications and Readmissions ("Evolution of DRGs," 2014).

Regardless of what method you use, it is wise to have some Adjustment for Resource Use to estimate Efficiency and Risk of Mortality. If your budget is really tight, you can start by using CMS's MS-DRGs for Severity/Resource Adjustment. In this situation, you will still have the challenge of Mortality Adjustment, which will be important for high Volume, high Acuity providers, such as Hospitalists.

A final note about cost

As we mentioned in the call-out box at the beginning of this chapter, when you are done shopping for your data, you will need to go through the check out line and pay the cashier. Keep this in mind as you shop. Some data may be available, but it may require special expertise to put in a form you can use for profiles. Some measures may be excellent, but their data collection may be difficult, perhaps requiring follow-up phone calls to patients, or large surveys – which are quite expensive, especially if continued over time. Keep track of your budget; you want good data, but at a good price.

Summary

In this chapter, we have covered potential data sources, including administrative data, cost accounting and provider billing datasets, quality management systems, niche specialty datasets that may reside within specialties, and specialty-oriented cooperative reporting projects.

Once you know where your data is and begin to review it, be sure measures are Valid, and that the stream of data is Accurate and Reliable. Further, address the need to Risk Adjust the data, especially for Severity (Resource Use) and Mortality. Finally, keep an eye on your budget to be sure you can afford everything you have put in your basket.

The next chapter will provide guidance on how to build your team, and integrate your profiling work into the quality fabric of your organization.

Reference List:

"About NQRN." (2015) AMA: American Medical Association. Retrieved from http://www.ama-assn.org/ama/pub/physician-resources/physician-consortium-performance-improvement/nqrn.page

"About the NUBC." (2014). National Uniform Billing Committee, American Hospital Association. Retrieved from http://www.nubc.org/aboutus/index.dhtml

Azoulay, A., Doris, N.M., Filion, K.B., Caron, J., Pilote, L., & Eisenberg, M.J. (2007). The use of the transition cost accounting system in health services research. *Cost Effectiveness and Resource Allocation : C/E, 5*, 11. doi:10.1186/1478-7547-5-11.

"Code sets." (2014). Centers for Medicare & Medicaid Services. Retrieved from http://www.cms.gov/Regulations-and-Guidance/HIPAA-Administrative-Simplification/TransactionCodeSetsStands/CodeSets.html

"Key points of the UB-04 (updated)." (2014). AHIMA: HIM Body of Knowledge. Retrieved from http://library.ahima.org/xpedio/groups/public/documents/ahima/bok1_047262.hcsp?dDocName=bok1_047262

Last, J.M. (Ed.) (2001). *A dictionary of epidemiology. (4th ed)*. New York: Oxford University Press.

Michelson, D. (2014). 10 reasons why hospitals are shifting to advanced cost accounting. Becker's Hospital CEO. Retrieved from http://www.beckershospital-review.com/finance/10-reasons-why-hospitals-are-shifting-to-advanced-cost-accounting.html

"National clinical registry inventory." (2014). American Medical Association. Retrieved from https://download.ama-assn.org/resources/doc/cqi/x-pub/nqrn-national-clinical-registry-inventory.pdf

Sanja, M.M. (2013). Impact of enterprise resource planning system in healthcare. *International Journal of Academic Research in Business and Social Services, (3)*. Retrieved from http://hrmars.com/hrmars_papers/Impact_of_Enterprise_Resource_Planning_System_in_Health_Care.pdf

"STS National Database." (2014). The Society of Thoracic Surgeons. Retrieved from http://www.sts.org/national-database

"The evolution of DRGs (updated)." (2014). AHIMA: HIM Body of Knowledge. Retrieved from http://library.ahima.org/xpedio/groups/public/documents/ahima/bok1_047260.hcsp?dDocName=bok1_047260

Torrey, T. (2015). What are CPT codes? About health. Retrieved from http://patients.about.com/od/costsconsumerism/a/cptcodes.htm

Trochim, W.M. (2006). Measurement validity types. Research Methods Knowledge Base. Retrieved from http://www.socialresearchmethods.net/kb/measval.php

NOTES

NOTES

Chapter 7

Getting the Kitchen Running:
How to Build Your Team

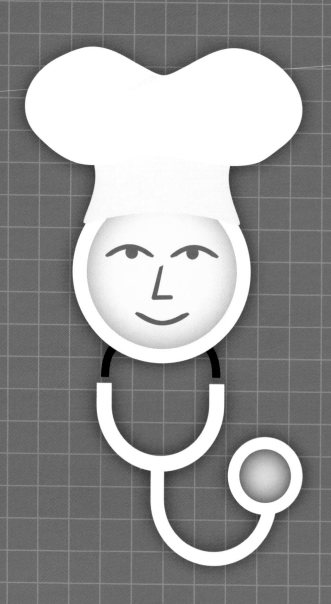

Kitchen Workflow

So far, we have covered planning menus, shopping for the right ingredients, preparing for the tasks before us, and cooking. But what is the best way to really make all this happen? This chapter addresses best practice in your kitchen: how to put your team together, achieve your goals, and make this a sustainable process. Remember that this is not a one-time banquet you are preparing, but rather a series of meals that need to be prepared and served in a sustainable fashion. Each meal should meet your diners' needs and be a little bit better than the last one.

Hopefully, you have physician help in the kitchen already; if not, go ahead and invite them in, remembering that provider profiling is by and for the Medical Staff. Yes, they tend to make a mess, and sometimes throw strange things together, but sharing the kitchen with them will help you and your team gain acceptance of your offerings. At the same time, they'll help you to come up with new items you may have never considered.

In many ways, this chapter is the most important part of the whole book. We have debated whether it should be the first chapter, or the last, and finally decided to keep it near the end; we add the advice that this chapter can be read first, last, or anywhere in between.

The process of developing profiles is not a "one and done" affair, with a beginning and an end; rather, it is a journey with a beginning followed by multiple way points, places to pause along the long trail to take stock and plan for the next leg of the journey. Going back to the kitchen, this is not a one-time gala dinner; rather, it is a full time kitchen, or, as we know it in the Southwest, a chuck wagon. The chuck wagon rides with the herd, and is always there to support the cattle drive. In a similar fashion, the team that builds and maintains profiles is always there to help providers perform better.

A solid, productive team is necessary for this work, so start by creating a team that includes members from Medical Staff leadership, the Medical Staff Office, the Quality Improvement and Safety Departments, Health Information (to include a coder/abstractor), and the Information Technology Department, including staff members who have been working on your electronic medical record. Be inclusive, ensuring you involve whoever is currently doing this work. This team will have a long and productive life, though its members and the nature of its work will change over time as the needs and the status of the process change. With this in mind, let's look at the team in more detail.

Building the Team

Medical Staff: Provider profiling is by and for the Medical Staff, and the ease of adoption will vary with its members participation in the process. The lead physician on this team should be a senior member of the Medical Staff with responsibility and authority for provider profiling. This may be the Chief of Staff, a past Chief of Staff, or the Physician Chair of Safety and/ or Quality. Invite senior clinical leaders who are willing to take the lead on profiles, including being willing to test metrics on their own performance, sharing them with the rest of the Medical Staff. These physicians may be senior clinicians, still in practice, who have been high volume providers in the past, or they may be present or former department or division heads. A former Chief of Staff who meets these criteria would be an ideal team member. These leaders will be your cadre of stalwarts to help both with profile construction, and promotion of the profiles to their peers, saying, "This is my profile, and I think it is helpful."

In your search for physician leaders, look for those who are matched with specific roles you need. For example, for leadership in the use of software-based profiling, look for clinicians who are tech savvy – these may be younger than your senior leaders, individuals who are comfortable with using computers and software applications, and can help "detail" the profiles internally. These leaders may also help you vet and gain support for any IT systems you use for data retrieval, analysis, and review. If you have recently adopted an electronic medical record, or are in the process of doing so, enlist a physician leader from that team to participate on the profiling initiative to share knowledge and process content.

Finally, look for leaders of the Advanced Practice Clinicians group to help with the construction of their unique profiles, and gain support of their peers. Consider running development work on these profiles in the background as you do the step-wise work outlined earlier, in Chapters 2, 3, and 4.

Medical Staff Office: Although many Medical Staffs carefully divide provider performance review and profiling from the Medical Staff Office functions, it is essential that the Medical Staff Office professionals be actively involved with profile construction and maintenance, both in support of the Medical Staff, and as customers of the process. Again, look to your Medical Staff bylaws, rules, and regulations for how performance data in profiles makes its way into the provider's file, and how it is used at the time of reappointment. Use this opportunity to update your processes as needed.

Quality Improvement and Safety: The department names may vary, but the leaders and staff responsible for Quality and Safety are essential elements of the provider profiling process, and in some organizations bear prime responsibility for these and related tasks. Most of the metrics that are used on provider profiles are also part of the broader organization's performance improvement work, so strive to align profile metrics with ongoing performance improvement projects. Doing so is not only efficient, but it also mainstreams the profiles into the broader work of the hospital, taking the profiling process into "prime time" and avoiding the impression that it is a niche activity or function required by regulatory bodies. These individuals will have insight into current quality challenges and areas where improvement is needed. Their knowledge and perspective is vital.

Health Information: Also known as "Medical Records," Health Information is responsible for the abstraction and coding of all records at discharge, as well as any concurrent coding done before discharge. The department is staffed by highly trained professionals whose jobs are to be sure the correct diagnosis and procedure codes are assigned based on chart documentation. Most of the metrics on profiles are based on the administrative (UB-04) data generated by this process; the value of this data is directly tied to the coding/abstracting processes and the quality of the chart documentation. Good communication among Health Information, Quality/Safety, and the Medical Staff is essential both in selecting metrics at the outset, and also in the ongoing maintenance of data. Understanding how codes are assigned and how they can change over time is essential in generating and maintaining valid profiles. It is not unusual for coding conventions to change in response to modifications in billing standards; thorough knowledge of these changes is essential to maintain reliable metrics.

At first, Health Information may not be identified as a potential contributor for provider profiling tasks. However, the professionals in this department have the unique experience of analyzing paper and electronic medical documentation, ensuring that it is coded appropriately ("Key responsibilities," 2015). These team members may have insight into areas of challenge and success, which are invaluable.

Information Technology: Most of the data used in profiles starts with the patient's medical record, which is dependent on provider documentation, and flows to Health Information. Abstraction and coding leads to the creation of the administrative dataset. At that point, the data is held in one or more databases; often, these are accessed by or function as part of multiple software systems. From these systems come the files or reports that feed the profiles, which are themselves likely part of a software system. Add to this the reality that a large percentage of charts are now electronic. Thus, it is clear that representation and support from your Information Technology Department is essential for the provider profiling processes to run smoothly. Be sure you have IT leadership on your team, and sufficient resources within the IT Department to support your work.

Your IT team members may also know of data stores that are unknown to others. They see not only the 'big picture' of the hospital's IT functioning, but also see the pieces that may not be immediately evident to others.

As you bring the full team together, consider designating a subset of team members, probably no more than 3, as an executive core team who can meet, either in person or remotely, on short notice to address any day-to-day issues that occur between regularly scheduled team meetings. Although the team is running on behalf of the Medical Staff, it is best to run its processes as a business line of the hospital, rather than a committee of the Medical Staff. In this way, you will get things done faster. It should be understood that the executive core team is not making decisions affecting major content or direction without the rest of the team, and that the core team always notifies the whole team when it meets or acts.

First Meeting

At your first team meeting, create a mission statement to broadly define the work of the team, emphasizing the necessity of support over time for the ongoing process. Don't spend a lot of time on this statement at the first meeting, as it can be modified as you go along, but define what you will be doing at the outset. There are a number of resources available to help with the creation of a mission statement ("Department/team performance," 2015). The following is offered as an example for illustration:

> *The Provider Profiling Team will continuously add value to [our organization] through the creation and maintenance of professional practice profiles for all providers, providing a tool for the Medical Staff to improve care processes and safety.*

In addition to a general mission statement, you can go further, creating a more detailed charter, which defines the purpose, importance, scope, deliverables, measures of success, and resources for the team (Scholtes et. al, 2010). Within this charter, you will visualize the final processes and products. Once you understand your goals, it is easier to achieve them. As our colleague Dr. Christopher Heller used to say, "You cannot get there from here, but you can get here from there." With an outcome defined, you can work backward to determine what has to be done to create it while establishing reasonable timeframes for completion. The charter should include what the profiles should look like and achieve, detailing all the reasons for doing them, the least of which should be regulatory demands. Look to the profiling and reporting process as a part of the continuing quest to improve care for all the patients served, consistent with the IOM's 6 aims, providing patient centered care that is: Safe, Effective, Efficient, Personalized, Timely, and Equitable ("Committee on quality health," 2001).

A sample charter based on an outline in *The Team Handbook* (Scholtes et. al, 2010) is offered here as an illustration. Free copies of *Team Handbook* worksheets can be downloaded from the Oriel website at www.teamhandbook.com.

Sample Team Charter: *(For illustration only)*

Purpose:
In partnership with the Medical Staff, design, create, and maintain provider profiles to meet or exceed the needs of both the Medical Staff and accrediting organizations.

Importance:
Provider profiles are a requirement of [accrediting organization] and an essential tool to help members of the Medical Staff and their departments understand and improve their performance in patient care and their citizenship as members of the Medical Staff.

Scope:
The team is responsible for the design, creation, and maintenance of professional practice profiles for members of the Medical Staff on a continuous basis, going forward with no set end point. The team will work in partnership with the Medical Staff Office, the Departments of Quality Improvement and Safety, Health Information, and Information Technology, with access to whatever resources are needed to meet the team's deliverables.

Deliverables:
The Generic Profile for all Medical Staff members with privileges will be completed and approved by the Medical Staff on or before [date], tested by at least 3 Medical Staff members by [date], and in production on or before [date]. Professional Practice Profiles for Pathology and Radiology will be completed by [date], for the Emergency Department by [date], and for Anesthesiology by [date]. The Chair of the team will create quarterly reports to be delivered to the Chief of Staff on the last day of the second month of each calendar quarter, to be presented by him or her to the Board of Trustees at the quarterly meeting the following month.

Measures:
The progress of the team will be tracked based on meeting established deliverables, detailed above.

Resources:
This team is responsible to the Chief of Staff [name] and VP of Hospital Administration [name]. Members of the team include the Chief of Staff [name], Chair of Quality and Safety [name], Director of Health Information [name], Director of the Medical Staff Office [name], and VP of Information Technology [name]. Hospital Administration and the Medical Staff shall provide whatever resources are needed to meet the team's deliverables within the defined scope, above.

One of the first tasks of the team is to review the current processes related to credentialing and privileging, along with your Medical Staff bylaws, rules, and regulations, to ensure that the latter are current and up-to-date, and that they provide the foundation for the profiles. Make a list of what is missing, agreeing upon a schedule to efficiently address what is needed.

Be sure you know how FPPE is triggered, and how these triggers may arise from OPPE profile reviews. At the time of an accreditation survey, this is a common question; therefore, you need to clearly define what practice variations on a profile will or will not trigger FPPE. For instance, the Medical Staff may determine that malpractice lawsuits, sentinel events, or specific validated incident reports trigger FPPE; however, you may wish to examine the defined triggers to ensure they are complete, up-to-date, and reflective of your hospital's processes. Check with your accreditation organization for more details and prescribed requirements; for example, HFAP specifies that, as of January 1, 2015, FPPE must include, among other things, identification of issues that impact the provision of safe, high quality care ("New OPPE/FPPE," 2014).

Perform an assessment of all major performance improvement projects underway within the organization. See how you can mesh the goals of these projects and initiatives with those associated with the profiles. For example, can the work of your team support performance measures for other project's performance, or can some of the metrics coming from PI projects be used for provider profiles?

Do a survey of all the data sources in the organization that can be used for metrics. For details, see Chapter 6 about data, its qualities, and its importance. Enlist the support of your IT Department; they know "where the data is buried."

Set expectations, goals, and a schedule of deliverables. Establish the waypoints in advance, and keep to that schedule. Dates to prioritize may include your next accreditation survey as well as any organizational deadlines that may influence the work of the team. Remember that multiple processes can run in parallel; an example of this is the design of profiles for Advanced Practice Clinicians. This project could be done by a subgroup as the main team works on the Generic Profile and advanced specialty profiles.

As you begin to build the profiles, mock them up as drafts (see call-out box on drafts in Chapter 1, p. 17), and have designated staff take them to the physician leaders of departments and/or divisions, requesting that they revise, add, or change as appropriate. Expect your providers to be critical, but realize that even the most scathing review usually ends with a positive suggestion that helps build that specialty's indicators; in time, you will find that these exchanges create broader support for the process.

As suggested earlier, certain members of the team should be tasked with promoting the profiles internally, which has been termed "academic detailing" (see call-out box, this page). This task involves using the same techniques that drug companies use to detail their newest offerings; in this case, the products are the profiles themselves. Part of this promotion includes having key senior leaders share their own profiles with their peers, discussing the value of the metrics, and the results as applied to a high volume provider.

Academic Detailing:

Simply put, academic detailing is a method of delivering new information to healthcare professionals via face-to-face educational interactions. The 'detailer' is typically also a healthcare professional, so the interchange is one of peer to peer. Historical focuses of academic detailing programs have been to change prescribing patterns for indicated medications, and to help providers adhere to medication guidelines associated with Diabetes Care (Patel, 2011).

Academic detailing is also described as a service that includes relationship-building, and is message-focused (Popish, 2013).

As you develop profiles and their included measures, don't forget to include metrics that will indicate the success of this process. Further, you will note the benefit of including relevant basic metrics, such as when milestones were reached, and if they were reached on time. Other metrics to consider include the percentage of Medical Staff members with completed, "live" profiles, and the percentage of the patient population covered by these clinicians. Additional related measures may include how often providers look at their own profiles and provider satisfaction surveys associated with the profiles and the profiling process.

Finally, do not outrun yourselves; take it slowly at first, but be methodical. Keep going and accelerate the pace as you progress, benefiting from success as it occurs. Keep an eye on the charter and look for more ways for the profiling concept to connect to and align with other parts and practices of the organization.

For some tips on running meetings, see Simple Rules for Running a Meeting, below.

Simple Rules for Running a Meeting:

- There is a leader who, like a host of a good news program, keeps track of the time and the agenda, and listens more than talks.
- Support the leader, who creates an agenda, has everyone agree to it, and follows it.
- Understand the importance of starting and ending on time.
- Remember: only one person talks at a time.
- If an important issues arises that requires more time, the leader will direct the group as it pauses to make a conscious decision to either revise the agenda to accommodate it or to schedule a separate meeting.
- Notice how the leader ends each meeting with a list of actionable items and deliverables; and shares the time and date of the next meeting.
- Within 24 hours, the leader writes up a summary of the meeting with the main points and assignments, and sends it to everyone via e-mail. He or she asks for any additions, deletions, or corrections with 72 hours. If none, understand that the leader will assume that everyone is in agreement with the summary.

Make sure that you only meet when productive work needs to be done, meaning decision-making and setting directions. Meet only as long as it takes to get the work done. Meet in-person at the start, and periodically thereafter, using web and phone conferencing in between meetings to minimize travel and improve efficiency.

◼ Summary

In this chapter, we discussed the value associated with building an interdisciplinary team to take on provider profiling as a continuous process integrated into the fabric of your organizational performance improvement plan. We highlighted how this process as a whole will bring value to the organization by supporting the IOM's 6 aims, providing patient centered care that is: Safe, Effective, Efficient, Personalized, Timely, and Equitable ("Committee on quality health," 2001). We provided guidance on writing both a mission statement and a charter to help reach these goals.

Reference List:

"Committee on quality health care in America, Institute of Medicine." (2001). *Crossing the Quality Chasm: A New Health System for the 21st Century.* Washington, DC: National Academy Press 41-56.

"Department/team performance management" (2015). Missionstatements.com. Retrieved from http://www.missionstatements.com/team_mission_statements.html

"Key responsibilities of health information." (2015). Peninsula Regional Medical Center. Retrieved from http://www.peninsula.org/KeyResponsibilitiesofHealth-Information

"New OPPE/FPPE standards – 2014 CAH manual." (2014). Healthcare Facilities Accreditation Program. Retrieved from http://www.hfap.org/blog/?p=9781

Patel, B. (2011). Back to school: Quality improvement through academic detailing. American Health and Drug Benefits. Retrieved from http://www.ahdbonline.com/issues/2011/november-december-2011-vol-4-no-7/872-article-872

Popish, S.J. (2013). Academic detailing: Using clinical evidence to improve care. Mental Health Clinician. Retrieved from http://cpnp.org/resource/mhc/2013/06/academic-detailing-using-clinical-evidence-improve-care

Scholtes, P.R., Joiner, B.L., & Streibel, B.J. (2010). The Team Handbook, Third Edition. Oriel STAT A MATRIX. Retrieved from http://www.orielstat.com/book/the-team-handbook-third-edition

"Team handbook worksheets." (2015). Oriel STAT A MATRIX. Retrieved from http://www.orielstat.com/cpages.aspx?mpgid=44&pgid=48

NOTES

Chapter 8

From Soup to Nuts: Putting It All Together

Bringing It All Together...

The kitchen is busy creating great meals for all the members of the Medical Staff, physicians and Advanced Practice Clinicians alike.

Let's pause to celebrate our success in all the great work we have done: putting together the best team with leadership from the Medical Staff; building menus to meet all our diners' needs, including those hard to cook for groups - Pathology, Radiology, Emergency Medicine, and Anesthesiology; shopping for just the right ingredients from the right stores; preparing our menu items carefully in terms of presentation, while working to make each day's offering just a little bit better than yesterday's. And we haven't forgotten those accrediting organizations that drop in from time to time to inspect the kitchen. We know they will be impressed with the kitchen and rave about our meals!

It is time to review our journey in the quest for provider excellence. Let's take a look at our path.

In the Preface, we reviewed terminology, deciding that, in this volume, we will be building *Professional Practice Profiles* supporting *Professional Practice Evaluation*, for all licensed independent practitioners, knowing that we may decide to name the profiles differently at the discretion of the Medical Staff.

In the Introduction, we answered 3 questions. First, we replied to the inquiry of "why build profiles?" Our answer was straightforward: to improve the performance of all providers with privileges, and to meet or exceed the requirements of our accrediting organizations, with special focus on the Joint Commission's requirements for Ongoing Professional Practice Evaluation (OPPE). Next, we addressed the question, "who do we profile?" Once again, our answer was straightforward: all licensed independent practitioners who are otherwise not properly evaluated through a human resources system. Finally, we asked, "what do we profile?" Our response was likewise direct: the privileges that each provider has, asking ourselves 4 questions: what does the provider have privileges to do? Is she doing it? Is she doing it well? (Smith & Pelletier, 2009). And, finally, should she have done it?

In Chapter 1, we went into more depth on who our customers are, what they expect of our profiles, how the profiles can be formatted, and how many profiles we need to build. Although our primary customers are the Medical Staff members, we cannot ignore licensing and accrediting bodies. At the time of this writing, 4 organizations accredit hospitals in the United States, conveying deemed status to facilities as CMS providers: The Joint Commission (TJC), Det Norske Veritas-Germanischer Lloyd Healthcare (DNV-GL Healthcare), the Healthcare Facilities Accreditation Program (HFAP), and the Center for Improvement in Healthcare Quality (CIHQ). TJC and HFAP standards for OPPE are almost identical, with DNV-GL very similar in terms of a profile cycle less than a year, with CIHQ echoing the basic CMS standards, requiring review only with the 2-year reappointment cycle.

We offered several choices for formatting profiles, beginning with TJC's recommended format patterned after the 6 competencies defined by the Accreditation Council for Graduate Medical Education (ACGME), then a format developed by the American Association for Physician Leadership (formerly the American College of Physician Executives), and adopted by The Greeley Company for use by Medical Staffs (Marder et al., 2007). We then offered our own third format, named Talis Qualis (TQ), meaning 'just as such,' as an alternative, with mapping to the ACGME 6 competencies. TQ is a start, a proposed format intended to grow and develop with your organizational needs and demands.

Chapter 1 concluded with a consideration of a number of distinct profiles you may need. We recommended a base Generic Profile, with added metrics for Surgical/Interventional providers and Internists, Hospitalists, and Pediatric providers. We went on to add profiles for 4 distinct specialties that require special attention both for measure construction and data sources; these we identified as Pathology, Radiology, Emergency Medicine, and Anesthesiology.

In Chapter 2, we built a provider profile using the base Generic Profile as an example, displayed in TQ format, with mapping to the ACGME format. We covered the basics of the profile's metrics: Volume, Acuity, Clinical Outcomes, Efficiency, Processes of Care, Patient Satisfaction, Citizenship, and Reviews. We discussed ways to adjust for Severity of Illness and Risk of Mortality. Further, we addressed measuring Complications based on administrative data, including use of 3 AHRQ modules: the Inpatient Quality Indicators

(IQIs), the Patient Safety Indicators (PSIs), and the Pediatric Quality Indicators (PDIs). In addition, we noted that Complication measures may be included with the help of the POA/NPOA flag, present on each secondary discharge diagnosis since 2007, as mandated by the Deficit Reduction Act of 2005 (DRA) ("Hospital-acquired conditions," 2014). We covered the challenges of provider attribution and reviewed the measurement of Efficiency using Cost of Care measures. Further, we noted that Processes of Care may be measured by TJC and CMS Core Measures, now known as an inclusive group that contains Joint Commission measures, Hospital Inpatient Quality Reporting Program measures (HIQR), and Hospital Outpatient Quality Reporting Program measures (HOQR). See Table 2.6 for a current list of these measures.

We finished up the Generic Profile build in Chapter 2 with Patient Satisfaction, Citizenship, and Review, discussing some of the issues that need to be considered when building any profile. Once we had the Generic Profile built, we showed how selected Outcome and Processes of Care metrics could be added for Surgeons/Proceduralists, and for Internists, Hospitalists, Pediatricians, and Family Medicine providers.

In Chapter 3, we started with the Generic foundation built in Chapter 2, adding metrics based on provider-specific privileges, reporting Volume, Acuity, Clinical Outcomes, Efficiency, and Processes of Care for each selected high volume, high risk, or problem-prone privilege, using the specialty of Gastroenterology as an example. We then walked through a prioritization method where we outlined how you can find your hospital's high volume, high risk, and problem-prone services, and rank them in order to guide your early work, looking for the small percent of privileges that cover the majority of your patient population. We illustrated how, once you have achieved this goal, you may continue to add privileges by specialty systematically, until all providers have privilege-specific profiles. We offered sample profiles for 9 top hospital specialties, ranked in descending order of estimated volume for a large community hospital.

In Chapter 4, we addressed "the Big Four," high volume specialties that are essential for the running of a hospital, but cannot be profiled based on a hospital discharge dataset: Pathology, Radiology, Emergency Medicine, and Anesthesiology. We considered each of the these specialties, noting that Pathology, Radiology, and Emergency Medicine are all services where short turn-around times and fast throughput are important measures of performance. Data sources were suggested, including provider billing systems; sample profiles were offered as draft starting points.

In Chapter 5, we completed our profile inventory by adding those non-physician providers, the Advanced Practice Clinicians (APCs), who must have profiles created, maintained, and reviewed as part of the Medical Staff OPPE process. We reviewed 4 common APC subgroups: Certified Registered Nurse Anesthetists (CRNAs); Certified Nurse Midwives (CNMs); Nurse Practitioners (NPs); and Physician Assistants (PAs). We offered sample privilege lists as reference points, and draft profiles for each of these 4 sub-groups.

Once we covered the full range of profiles needed, Chapter 6 took us shopping for data, checking our purchases for Validity, Accuracy, and Reliability, and ensuring we maintained our budget. We reviewed common data sources, with a discussion of the standard billing format approved by the National Uniform Billing Committee (NUBC), UB-04, also known as "administrative data" ("About the NUBC," 2014). We discussed other data sources, including hospital-specific cost accounting systems, CPT-based provider billing systems, and care management/case management/quality/safety/risk systems. We also noted that specialty datasets residing in procedural settings, including the OR, may be a rich source of procedure-specific metrics. In addition, we highlighted how many subspecialties maintain cooperative databases, which may provide both specialty-specific metrics as well as comparative data. A list of these datasets is maintained by the AMA as part of the National Quality Registry Network (NQRN) ("About NQRN," 2014). A short list of these databases relevant to provider profiles was provided at the end of Chapter 6.

As we began with Chapter 7, we noted how it was perhaps the most important chapter of all. Therein, we described building the team that will make all this happen. We suggested you start by finding team members representing the Medical Staff, your most important customers, as well as representatives from the Medical Staff Office, Quality Improvement, Safety, Health Information, and Information Technology. We recommend that, at your first meeting, you create a mission statement and a team charter to help define and guide your work going forward (Scholtes, Joiner, & Streibel, 2010). As an example, we provided a sample mission statement and team charter. Early key steps for the team were outlined, including a review of the current Medical Staff bylaws, rules, and regulations. Further, we put forward our experience-based proposal that you perform an assessment of all major performance improvement projects currently underway in your hospital, looking for possible integration of initiatives with the provider profiles. We went on to suggest that you set team expectations, goals, and a schedule of deliverables, and plan how the profiles will be rolled out and promoted internally through academic detailing (Popish, 2013).

That's it! We hope you have found our kitchen tour helpful and enjoyable. Now, get out the pots and pans and let's get started on our journey, providing tasty meals and fine nutrition in a continuous process by and for the Medical Staff, to provide patient-centered care that is Safe, Effective, Efficient, Personalized, Timely, and Equitable ("Committee on quality health," 2001). Once you start cooking, you will be creating *Data-Driven Healthcare Improvement* in your organization, and perfecting your own *Recipe for Provider Excellence.*

Reference List:

"About NQRN." (2015). American Medical Association. Retrieved from http://www.ama-assn.org/ama/pub/physician-resources/physician-consortium-performance-improvement/nqrn.page

"About the NUBC." (2014). National Uniform Billing Committee, American Hospital Association. Retrieved from http://www.nubc.org/aboutus/index.dhtml

"Committee on quality health care in America, Institute of Medicine." (2001). *Crossing the Quality Chasm: A New Health System for the 21st Century,* Washington, DC: National Academy Press, 41-56.

"Hospital-acquired conditions (present on admission indicator)." (2014). Centers for Medicare and Medicaid Services. Retrieved from http://www.cms.gov/Medicare/Medicare-Fee-for-Service-Payment/HospitalAcqCond/index.html?redirect=/HospitalAcqCond/02_Statute_Regulations_Program_Instructions.asp#TopOfPage

Marder, R., Smith, M., Smith, M., & Searcy, V. (2007). *Measuring physician competency, how to collect, assess, and provide performance data. (2nd edition).* Marblehead, MA: HCPro, Inc.

Popish, S.J. (2013). Academic detailing: Using clinical evidence to improve care. Mental Health Clinician. Retrieved from http://cpnp.org/resource/mhc/2013/06/academic-detailing-using-clinical-evidence-improve-care

Scholtes, P.R., Joiner, B.L., & Streibel, B.J. (2010). *The Team Handbook, Third Edition.* Oriel STAT A MATRIX, Edison, NJ.

Smith, M.A. & Pelletier, S. (2009). *Assessing the competency of low-volume practitioners.* HCPro: Marblehead, MA.

NOTES

Glossary

The intention of this Glossary is to provide brief definitions and introductions to terms and phrases used throughout this text. Every effort has been made to ensure this listing includes as many of the terms and phrases used that may be unfamiliar; at the same time, many of the inclusions may be quite familiar to you, but perhaps not to all readers. Note that many of the items included herein are given due diligence within the chapters of the text itself; therefore, please reference the text for more information and insight, as needed. If you are seeking even more information, we encourage you to access any of the relevant references included at the end of this glossary listing and each chapter. Note that the terms in italics are either unique to this text, or defined here in a way that is unique.

TERM	DEFINITION
Academic Detailing	With roots in the peer-to-peer sharing of pharmaceutical best practice and insights into the use of new or different medications to address patient needs, Academic Detailing includes building a relationship and providing message-focused information to clinicians (Popish, 2013).
Accreditation Council for Graduate Medical Education	(ACGME) A private professional organization responsible for the accreditation of ~9,500 residency education programs in the United States, the ACGME accredits residency programs in 140 specialty and subspecialty areas of Medicine, including all programs leading to primary Board Certification of the 24 member boards of the American Board of Medical Specialties ("About ACGME," 2015).
Accuracy	The degree to which a measurement or an estimate based on measurements represents the true value of the attribute that is being measured is termed Accuracy (Porta, 2014).
Advanced Practice Clinician	(APC) The term *Advanced Practice Clinician* encompasses all non-physician providers who can practice independently. In this text, APCs include Certified Registered Nurse Anesthetists (CRNAs), Certified Nurse Midwives (CNMs), Nurse Practitioners (NPs), and Physician Assistants (PAs). Other terms used outside of this text for this group of providers include "mid-level providers," "allied health providers/practitioners," "physician extenders," "non-physician providers," and "limited license providers."

TERM	DEFINITION
Agency for Healthcare Research and Quality	(AHRQ) As part of the US Department of Health and Human Services, the AHRQ seeks to promote evidence-based healthcare quality and outcomes. In 1994, the AHRQ created a set of quality measures that used hospital administrative data provided by the Healthcare Cost and Utilization Project (HCUP) to identify potential quality of care problems. In 1998, researchers at UCSF and the Stanford University Evidence-Based Practice Center revised the original set of measures to create the AHRQ QIs (Quality Indicators), originally provided in 2 modules, Prevention Quality Indicators (PQIs) and Inpatient Quality indicators (IQIs). By 2006, additional modules were added, Patient Safety Indicators (PSIs) and Pediatric Quality Indicators (PDIs) (Hughes, 2008). Of the 4 AHRQ QI modules, the IQIs, PSIs, and PDIs are viewed as the most applicable to measuring inpatient Quality and Complications of Care; see Tables 2.2, 2.3, 2.4.
All Patient Refined-Diagnosis-Related Group	(APR-DRG) This DRG method offers an advanced form of diagnostic-related groups developed by 3M in 1990 to address both Severity of Illness and Risk of Mortality for all patient populations. Each APR-DRG category assigns the patient to 1 of 4 subclasses for Severity of Illness, and for Risk of Mortality ("The evolution of DRGs," 2014).
American College of Surgeons	(ACS) The ACS is a scientific and educational association of Surgeons founded in 1913 to improve the quality of care for the surgical patient by setting standards for surgical education and practice. As of this writing, the College has more than 80,000 members, including more than 6,600 fellows in other countries, making it the largest organization of Surgeons in the world ("About ACS," 2015).
American Osteopathic Association/Healthcare Facility Accreditation Program	(AOA/HFAP) See Healthcare Facility Accreditation Program, below.
Average Length of Stay	(ALOS) Average Length of Stay is the sum of patient days (numerator) divided by the sum of discharged encounters (denominator). The day of admission is day 1.
Case Mix Index	(CMI) The average of MS-DRG Relative Weights, or other Severity/Acuity index, such as APR-DRG subclass weights, for a selected population, is the Case Mix Index. A Relative Weight (RW) is assigned to each MS-DRG to reflect the average hospital resource consumption by patients for that MS-DRG, relative to all patients. The CMI is a measure of the resources needed to care for a population of patients ("Calculation of," 2015).

TERM	DEFINITION
Center for Improvement in Healthcare Quality	(CIHQ) The Center for Improvement in Healthcare Quality is a membership-based organization comprised primarily of acute care and critical access hospitals, established in 1999, that advocates on behalf of its members to create an effective regulatory environment. CIHQ includes 3 divisions, Hospital Accreditation, Hospital Support, and Professional Certification ("About our organization," 2015).
Centers for Medicare and Medicaid Services	(CMS) CMS is a US government agency that runs the federal Medicare and Medicaid programs, which were originally enacted into law in 1965. Its comprehensive regulations impact the hospitals, payers, patients, and providers that participate in or seek care via its programs ("Regulations," 2015).
Clinical Quality Measures	(CQMs) CMS defines a set of measures, termed Clinical Quality Measures, to track the quality of health care services provided by eligible professionals, acute care hospitals, and critical access hospitals within the health care system. These measures are extensive and change over time. For details, the reader is encouraged to check the CMS website ("Clinical quality measures," 2015).
Conditions of Participation	(CoPs) Developed by CMS, the Conditions of Participation are the standards that health care organizations must meet to participate in Medicare and Medicaid programs. CoPs ensure quality services and protection of the health and safety of program beneficiaries ("Centers for Medicare," 2015).
Core Measures	Initially developed by The Joint Commission with input from clinical stakeholders in 1999, 4 core measurement areas for hospitals were announced in 2001, including acute myocardial infarction (AMI) and heart failure (HF). Simultaneously, TJC worked with CMS on the AMI and HF sets that were common to both organizations to create alignment of measure specifications. By November 2003, CMS and TJC aligned common measures, resulting in the Specifications Manual for National Hospital Inpatient Quality Measures to be used by both organizations ("Core measure sets," 2015).
Det Norske Veritas – Germanischer Lloyd Healthcare, Inc.	(DNV-GL Healthcare) This organization provides accreditation, certification, and training programs for hospitals. The accreditation arm, NIAHO, integrates ISO 9001 with the Medicare CoPs. It has been accrediting hospitals since 2008, working with almost 500 hospitals across the US as of this writing ("Hospital accreditation," 2015).

TERM	DEFINITION
Diagnostic Related Group	(DRG) Developed in the early 1970s at Yale University, the DRG methodology assigns a numeric value to an acute care inpatient hospital episode of care, which serves as a Relative Weight factor, intended to represent the resource intensity of hospital care of the clinical group classified to that specific DRG. As a reimbursement system, the DRG assignment determines the payment level the hospital will receive. In 1983, the Health Care Financing Administration (HCFA; now the Centers for Medicare and Medicaid Services) implemented DRGs for the Inpatient Prospective Payment System (IPPS). See also APR-DRG ("The evolution of DRGs," 2014).
Encounter	An episode of care with a beginning and an end is an Encounter. For inpatients, an Encounter is the same as an admission/discharge. For outpatients, it may be a single visit to the office or the Emergency Room. This term is commonly used in databases and IT systems.
Focused Professional Practice Evaluation	(FPPE) A standard of The Joint Commission, Focused Professional Practice Evaluation takes place at the time of initial appointment and privileging, when new privileges are requested, or when an event and/or data trend occurs, per Medical Staff rules, that warrants more focused evaluation of the provider's performance ("What are OPPE," 2014).
Generic Profile	In this text, we use the term Generic Profile to include the basic, starting profile that may later be fine-tuned to meet specific departmental or division needs. In the TQ format, the Generic Profile offers the first step on the path to developing the provider profiles that will meet your hospital's evaluative and reporting needs.
Get With The Guidelines	(GWTG) An American Heart Association/American Stroke Association in-hospital quality improvement program focused on Stroke, Heart Failure, AFIB, and Resuscitation, Get With The Guidelines helps hospitals receive recognition for meeting certain quality of care standards. GWTG certification helps hospitals meet requirements associated with data and improvement in quality of care ("Get With The Guidelines," 2015).
Healthcare Cost and Utilization Project	(HCUP) Sponsored by AHRQ, HCUP is the largest collection of national and state-specific hospital care databases, a partnership among federal, state, and industry entities. Its data begins in 1988 ("HCUP frequently," 2015).
Healthcare Facilities Accreditation Program	(HFAP) An accreditation organization with deeming authority by CMS, HFAP focuses on high quality patient care and safety by applying established standards of care. In 2009, more than 200 hospitals and 200 other healthcare facilities were accredited by HFAP (Meldi, Rhoades, & Gippe, 2009). This organization is also termed AOA/HFAP, indicating its relationship to the American Osteopathic Association.

TERM	DEFINITION
Hospital Acquired Conditions	(HACs) Hospital Acquired Conditions are a set of conditions as defined by CMS, acquired during a hospitalization, and deemed to be potentially preventable. Beginning in 2008, if a CMS-defined HAC caused the MS-DRG on a Medicare beneficiary to rise to a higher Relative Weight and therefore higher reimbursement under the IPPS, then, within parameters set by CMS, the MS-DRG would be rolled back to the MS-DRG with the lower RW. Thus, reimbursement for the admission would be lower ("Hospital acquired," 2015).
Hospital Consumer Assessment of Healthcare Providers and Systems	(HCAHPS) Developed by CMS, HCAHPS is a standardized survey of patients' perspectives on their hospital care. The publically reported results are intended to be used for comparison of hospitals on metrics that are important to consumers. A goal of HCAHPS is to enhance accountability by increasing the transparency of hospital quality care ("HCAHPS," 2014).
Hospital Inpatient Quality Reporting	(HIQR or IQR) Developed by CMS as a result of the Medicare Prescription Drug Improvement and Modernization Act (MMA) of 2003, this program provides healthcare consumers with the information they need to make informed healthcare choices. Hospitals report information, which is then made available via the Hospital Compare website. Data includes quality measures associated with common health conditions that result in inpatient admissions ("Hospital inpatient," 2015).
Hospital Outpatient Quality Reporting	(HOQR or OQR) Modeled after the HIQR program, the Outpatient Quality Reporting initiative supports quality data reporting for outpatient hospital services. Data reported on standardized measures allows hospitals to receive the full annual update to its Outpatient Prospective Payment System (OPPS) rate. It is a voluntary CMS program ("Hospital outpatient," 2015).
Hospital Quality Initiative	(HQI) HQI, a CMS initiative, provides information on quality of care and encourages providers to improve the quality of care they provide. Hospital Compare, which debuted in 2005, is a primary tool used for public reporting of valid, credible, user-friendly information ("Hospital quality," 2008).
Indicator	Synonymous with the terms *measure* and *metric*, Indicator types include counts, rates, percentages, and averages. Provider profiles consist of indicators grouped by category.

TERM	DEFINITION
Inpatient Prospective Payment System	(IPPS) Hospitals that contract with Medicare to furnish acute hospital inpatient care agree to accept payment on a per discharge or per case basis as determined by the IPPS, which assigns each patient a MS-DRG. The specific MS-DRG is associated with a pre-determined reimbursement amount. The reimbursement is calculated by multiplying the MS-DRG Relative Weight (RW) by the base rate. Base rates, calculated annually, are determined, in part, by the hospital's local wage index, with additional amounts added for hospitals engaged in teaching medical residents, treating a disproportionate share of low-income patients, addressing cases that involve certain approved new technologies, and high-cost outlier cases ("Acute care hospital inpatient," 2013).
Institute of Medicine	(IOM) The Institute of Medicine is the health arm of the National Academy of Sciences, chartered under President Abraham Lincoln in 1863. As an independent, nonprofit organization working outside of government, the IOM works to help those in government and the private sector make informed health decisions by providing evidence upon which they can rely. Many of the IOM studies begin as specific mandates from Congress; others are requested by federal agencies or independent organizations. The IOM also convenes a series of forums, roundtables, and standing committees to facilitate discussion, discovery, and critical cross-disciplinary thinking ("About the IOM," 2013).
International Classification of Diseases	(ICD) The International Classification of Diseases (ICD) is a standard taxonomy of diseases and health problems, maintained by the World Health Organization. It classifies diseases and other health problems recorded on many types of health and vital records, including death certificates. In addition to enabling the storage and retrieval of diagnostic information for clinical, epidemiological, and quality purposes, these records also provide the basis for the compilation of national mortality and morbidity statistics by WHO Member States. Finally, ICD is used for reimbursement and resource allocation decision-making by countries. All WHO Member States use the ICD, which has been translated into 43 languages. The current version in use in the United States is the ICD, Ninth Revision, Clinical Modification (ICD-9-CM); it acts as the official system for assigning codes to diagnoses and procedures associated with hospital utilization in the United States ("International classification," 2015). ICD-10 was endorsed by the 43rd World Health Assembly in May 1990 and came into use in WHO Member States starting in 1994. As of this writing, ICD-10 will become the new version in the United States, replacing ICD-9-CM, as of October 1, 2015 ("ICD-10," 2015).

TERM	DEFINITION
Medicare Severity-Diagnosis Related Groups	(MS-DRGs) See DRG.
National Integrated Accreditation for Healthcare Organizations	(NIAHO) See DNV-GL.
National Quality Registry Network	(NQRN) Run by the AMA, the NQRN is a national voluntary network of organizations operating clinical registries. The NQRN establishes and disseminates leading practices for registries, supports a learning network to accelerate registry development, growth, and use, and develops resources for the clinical registry industry ("About NQRN," 2015).
Not Present on Admission	(NPOA) A medical problem or condition may not be present at the time the order for inpatient admission occurs; if it is not, it is designated NPOA. NPOA includes conditions that develop during the inpatient encounter. CMS mandates POA/NPOA reporting for Medicare inpatient admissions ("Hospital-acquired," 2013).
Ongoing Professional Practice Evaluation	(OPPE) OPPE is a tool used to identify areas where improvement may be needed related to provider performance. It serves as a means of evaluating professional practice, provider competency, and quality of care delivered by providers, and supports the provision of objective data in decisions related to a provider's privileges and practice (Wise, 2013).
Outcomes	Outcomes are all the possible results that may stem from exposure to a causal factor or from preventative or therapeutic interventions. Outcomes include all identified changes in health status arising as a consequence of the handling of a health problem (Porta, 2014).
Pareto Principle	The Pareto Principle is the concept that 20 percent of a set of items is responsible for 80 percent of the outcome of interest. Based on the work of the Italian economist and sociologist Vilfredo Pareto in the early 1900's, it was developed into a management principle by Dr. Joseph M. Juran, bringing it into quality management as the Pareto Principle ("Pareto principle,"2005). Also called the 80:20 Rule, the Pareto Principle is used to analyze data. Juran applied the Pareto Principle to quality control and found that 80 percent of problems stem from 20 percent of possible causes ("Statistical process control," 2002).

TERM	DEFINITION
Physician Quality Reporting System	(PQRS) Formerly known as the Physician Quality Reporting Initiative (PQRI), PQRS is a program that uses incentive payments and negative payment adjustments to promote quality reporting information by eligible professionals for services covered by Physician Fee Schedule and services provided to Medicare Part B Fee-for-Service (FFS) beneficiaries ("Physician quality," 2015).
Present on Admission	(POA) Present on Admission indicates that a medical problem or condition was present at the time of inpatient admission; see NPOA.
Principal Procedure Provider	The provider who was the Surgeon/Proceduralist for the principal procedure during an inpatient encounter is the Principal Procedure Provider.
Reliability	The degree of stability exhibited when a measurement is repeated under identical conditions is termed Reliability (Porta, 2014).
Relative Weight	(RW) A weight that is assigned to each diagnosis related group (DRG) that reflects the average relative cost of a case in that group compared to the costs for an average Medicare case is the Relative Weight. The RW allows for the calculation of the Medicare Inpatient Prospective Payment System (IPPS) rate, which is intended to cover the average costs a provider incurs in the provision of care for one type of inpatient case as compared to another. The RWs are recalibrated annually, based on standard charges ("Payment system," 2009). See also Case Mix Index.
Risk Adjustment	Risk Adjustment acts as a corrective tool by adjusting the reported patient outcomes and variations associated with Risk among patients and patient groups. Risk Adjustment allows for the comparison of hospitals and providers by accounting for higher risk patients, including those who are sicker and those who have multiple comorbidities ("What is risk," 2014).
Talis Qualis	(TQ) *Talis Qualis* is the name of our proposed, alternate format for provider profiling, which, in Latin, means "just as such." We selected this name due to the intention of our format—it is a starting point from which you can make adjustments, revisions, and additions to ensure the profiling format meets your needs.

TERM	DEFINITION
The Joint Commission	(TJC) The Joint Commission provides accreditation and certification to more than 20,500 health care organizations and programs in the U.S. Its accreditation and certification is seen as a symbol of quality, illustrative of the entity's commitment to meeting established performance standards. Its mission includes a priority on evaluation and safety ("About The Joint Commission," 2015). Previous names include the Joint Commission on Accreditation of Hospitals (JCAH) and the Joint Commission on Accreditation of Healthcare Organizations (JCAHO) ("Mission and history," 2015).
UB-04	The standard, uniform bill (UB) for institutional healthcare providers that is used throughout the United States is called the UB-04. Its users include hospitals, nursing homes, hospices, home health agencies, insurance carriers, and others. Intended to provide a standardized form for billing across the healthcare spectrum, the UB-04 form has been in use since 2007 ("Definitions," 2014).
Validity	Validity expresses the degree to which a measurement measures what it purports to measure. Several types of Validity exist; these include: • Construct Validity: The extent to which the measurement corresponds to theoretical concepts or constructs concerning the phenomenon under study. For example, if, based on theoretical grounds, the measure should change with age, then a measure with Construct Validity should reflect a change with age. • Content Validity: The extent to which the measurement incorporates the domain of the phenomenon under study. For example, a measurement of functional health status should embrace activities of daily living (occupational, family, and social functioning, etc.). • Criterion Validity: The extent to which the measurement correlates with an external criterion of the phenomenon under study. • Face Validity: The extent to which a measurement appears reasonable on superficial inspection, on "the face of it." Note that although Face Validity is by definition the most superficial of these forms, it is important when seeking consensus among providers on profile measures. The measure should make sense (Last, 2001).

TERM	DEFINITION
Value-Based Purchasing	(VBP) The Hospital Value-Based Purchasing Program is a CMS initiative that rewards acute care hospitals with incentive payments based on either how well they perform on measures, or how much they improve their performance on each measure compared to the performance during a baseline period. Performance is based on an approved set of measures and dimensions, grouped into domains. For FY 2015, there are 4 domains: Clinical Processes of Care, Patient Experience of Care, Outcome, and Efficiency ("Hospital value-based purchasing," 2013).

Reference List:

"About ACGME." (2015) Accreditation Council for Graduate Medical Education. Retrieved from https://www.acgme.org/acgmeweb/tabid/116/About.aspx

"About ACS." (2015). American College of Surgeons. Retrieved from https://www.facs.org/about-acs

"About ICD-9 coding." (2015). American Hospital Association Central Office. Retrieved from http://www.ahacentraloffice.org/codes/ICD9.shtml

"About NQRN." (2015). American Medical Association. Retrieved from http://www.ama-assn.org/ama/pub/physician-resources/physician-consortium-performance-improvement/nqrn.page

"About our organization." (2015). Center for Improvement in Healthcare Quality. Retrieved from https://www.cihq.org/about_our_organization.asp

"About the IOM." (2013). Institute of Medicine of the National Academies. Retrieved from http://www.iom.edu/About-IOM.aspx

"About The Joint Commission." (2015). The Joint Commission. Retrieved from http://www.jointcommission.org/about_us/about_the_joint_commission_main.aspx

"Acute care hospital inpatient prospective payment system." (2013). Centers for Medicare & Medicaid Services. Retrieved from http://www.cms.gov/Outreach-and-Education/Medicare-Learning-NetworkMLN/MLNProducts/downloads/AcutePaymtSysfctsht.pdf

"Acute inpatient PPS." (2014). Centers for Medicare and Medicaid Services. Retrieved from http://www.cms.gov/Medicare/Medicare-Fee-for-Service-Payment/AcuteInpatientPPS/index.html?redirect=/acuteinpatientpps/

"Calculation of the Office of Statewide Health Planning and Development's (OSHPD) case mix index (CMI)." (2015). OSHPD. Retrieved from http://www.oshpd.ca.gov/HID/Products/PatDischargeData/CaseMixIndex/CMI/ExampleCalculation.pdf

"Centers for Medicare and Medicaid Services—conditions of participation." (2015). National Association of Clinical Nurse Specialists. Retrieved from http://www.nacns.org/html/participation.php

"Clinical quality measures basics." (2014). Centers for Medicare and Medicaid Services. Retrieved from http://www.cms.gov/Regulations-and-Guidance/Legislation/EHRIncentivePrograms/ClinicalQualityMeasures.html

"Core measure sets." (2015). The Joint Commission. Retrieved from http://www.jointcommission.org/core_measure_sets.aspx

"Definitions of the UB-04 form." (2014). UB04 Knowledge Trek, powered by BridgeFront. Retrieved from http://www.ub04.net/history_ub04_1.php

"Get With The Guidelines." (2015). American Heart Association. Retrieved from http://www.heart.org/HEARTORG/HealthcareResearch/HospitalAccreditationCertification/Get-With-The-Guidelines-Can-Help-Get-You-There-Faster_UCM_455447_SubHomePage.jsp

"HCAHPS: Patients' perspectives of care survey." (2014). Centers for Medicare and Medicaid Services. Retrieved from http://www.cms.gov/Medicare/Quality-Initiatives-Patient-Assessment-Instruments/HospitalQualityInits/HospitalHCAHPS.html

"HCUP frequently asked questions." (2015). Healthcare Cost and Utilization Project, AHRQ. Retrieved from http://www.hcup-us.ahrq.gov/tech_assist/faq.jsp#general

"Hospital accreditation." (2015). DNV-GL. Retrieved from http://dnvglhealthcare.com/accreditations/hospital-accreditation

"Hospital acquired conditions." (2015). US Department of Health and Human Services: Agency for Healthcare Research and Quality. Retrieved from http://www.guideline.gov/resources/hospital-acquired-conditions.aspx

"Hospital-acquired conditions and present on admission indicator reporting provision." (2013). Centers for Medicare and Medicaid Services, Medicare Learning Network. Retrieved from http://www.cms.gov/Outreach-and-Education/Medicare-Learning-Network-MLN/MLNProducts/downloads/wPOAFactSheet.pdf

"Hospital inpatient quality reporting (IQR) program overview." (2015). QualityNet. Retrieved from http://www.qualitynet.org/dcs Content-Server?cid=1138115987129&pagename=QnetPublic%2FPage%2FQnetTier2

"Hospital outpatient quality reporting (OQR) program overview." (2015). QualityNet. Retrieved from http://www.qualitynet.org/dcs/Content Server?cid=1191255879384&pagename=QnetPublic%2F-Page%2FQnetTier2&c=Page

"Hospital quality initiative overview." (2008). Centers for Medicare and Medicaid Services. Retrieved from http://www.cms.gov/Medicare/Quality-Initiatives-Patient-AssessmentInstruments/HospitalQualityInits/downloads/hospitaloverview.pdf

"Hospital value-based purchasing program." (2013). Department of Health and Human Services, Centers for Medicare & Medicaid Services. Retrieved from http://www.cms.gov/Outreach-and-Education/Medicare-Learning-Network-MLN/MLNProducts/downloads/Hospital_VBPurchasing_Fact_Sheet_ICN907664.pdf

Hughes RG, Ed. (2008). *Patient Safety and Quality: An evidence-Based Handbook for Nurses*. Rockville,MD: Agency for Healthcare Research and Quality. Retrieved from http://www.ncbi.nlm.nih.gov/books/NBK2651/

"ICD-10." (2015). Centers for Medicare and Medicaid Services. Retrieved from http://www.cms.gov/Medicare/Coding/ICD10/index.html?redirect=/icd10

"Inpatient quality indicators overview." (2014). Agency for Healthcare Research and Quality. Retrieved from http://www.qualityindicators.ahrq.gov/modules/iqi_overview.aspx

"International classification of diseases (ICD)." (2015). World Health Organization. Retrieved from http://www.who.int/classifications/icd/en/

Last, J.M. (Ed.) (2001). *A dictionary of epidemiology. (4th ed)*. New York: Oxford University Press.

Meldi, D., Rhoades, F., & Gippe, A. (2009). The big three: A side by side matrix comparing hospital accrediting agencies. Synergy. Retrieved from http://www.namss.org/Portals/0/Regulatory/The%20Big%20Three%20A%20Side%20by%20Side%20Matrix%20Comparing%20Hospital%20Accrediting%20Agencies.pdf

"Mission and history." (2015). Joint Commission Resources. Retrieved from http://www.jcrinc.com/about-jcr/mission-history/

"Patient safety indicators overview." (2014). Agency for Healthcare Research and Quality. Retrieved from http://www.qualityindicators.ahrq.gov/modules/psi_overview.aspx

"Payment system fact sheet series." (2009). Medicare Learning Network. Retrieved from http://www.ahd.com/AcutePaymtSysfctsht_JAN09.pdf

"Physician quality reporting system." (2015). Centers for Medicare and Medicaid Services. Retrieved from http://www.cms.gov/Medicare/Quality-Initiatives-Patient-Assessment-Instruments/PQRS/index.html?redirect=/PQRS/

Popish, S.J. (2013). Academic detailing: Using academic evidence to improve care. Mental Health Clinician. Retrieved from http://cpnp.org/resource/mhc/2013/06/academic-detailing-using-clinical-evidence-improve-care

Porta, M. (2014). *A Dictionary of Epidemiology*. New York: Oxford.

"Present on admission frequently asked questions." (2014). WellCare. Retrieved from https://www.wellcare.com/WCAssets/corporate/assets/Present_on_Admission_FAQs.pdf

"Regulations & guidance." (2015). Centers for Medicare and Medicaid Services. Retrieved from http://www.cms.gov/Regulations-and-Guidance/Regulations-and-Guidance.html

"Statistical process control, part 3: Pareto analysis and check sheets." (2002). Retrieved from http://owic.oregonstate.edu/sites/default/files/pubs/EM8771.pdf

"The evolution of DRGs (updated)." (2014). AHIMA: HIM Body of Knowledge. Retrieved from http://library.ahima.org/xpedio/groups/public/documents/ahima/bok1_047260.hcsp?dDocName=bok1_047260

"What are OPPE and FPPE?" (2014). College of American Pathologists. Retrieved from http://www.cap.org/apps/docs/reference/oppe_fppe.pdf

"What is risk adjustment?" (2014). The Society of Thoracic Surgeons. Retrieved from http://www.sts.org/patient-information/what-risk-adjustment

Wise, R.A. (2013). OPPE and FPPE: Tools to help make privileging decisions. Retrieved from http://www.jointcommission.org/jc_physician_blog/oppe_fppe_tools_privileging_decisions/

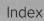
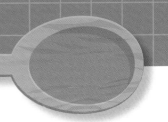

Index

Encounter 19, 22, 43, 45, 49, 100, 156, 193, 196, 197
Enterprise Resource Planning, ERP 157
Equitable 3, 175, 180, 187
Evalumetrics™ 102, 107
Evidence-Based 46, 47, 191

F
Face Validity 162, 198
Focused Professional Practice Evaluation, FPPE 3, 11, 24, 50, 101, 102, 107, 177, 180, 193, 202

G
Gastroenterologist 23, 71, 100
Gastroenterology 1, 27, 38, 70, 72, 74, 77, 107, 160, 185
General Practitioners 79
General Surgery 27, 62, 78, 79, 89
Generic Profile v, 6, 21, 25, 26, 42, 43, 45, 47, 49, 50, 51, 52, 53, 55, 57, 59, 61, 63, 65, 67, 69, 71, 73, 74, 80, 82, 157, 176, 177, 184, 185, 193
Get With The Guidelines, GWTG 159, 160, 193
Greeley, Greeley Model 9, 20, 184

H
Head and Neck Surgery 79
Healthcare Cost and Utilization Project, HCUP 46, 191, 193, 200
Healthcare Facilities Accreditation Program, HFAP 10, 12, 14, 15, 28, 32, 177, 184, 191, 193
Health Information 45, 53, 163, 171, 173, 174, 176, 186
Hospice 39, 44, 81
Hospital-Acquired Conditions, HACs 47, 53, 61, 185, 188, 194, 201
Hospital Consumer Assessment of Healthcare Providers and Systems, HCAHPS 55, 63, 194, 200
Hospital Inpatient Quality Reporting, HIQR 48, 185, 194
Hospitalist 25, 26, 38, 80, 83, 90
Hospital Medicine 79, 80, 90
Hospital Outpatient Quality Reporting, HOQR 48, 185, 194
Hospital Quality Initiative, HQI 194

I
ICU 43, 62, 65, 80, 91, 100, 126
Information Technology, IT 46, 105, 128, 158, 163, 164, 171, 172, 174, 176, 177, 186, 193
Inpatient Prospective Payment System, IPPS 193, 194, 195, 197
Inpatient Quality Indicators, IQIs 46, 53, 58, 184, 191, 201
Institute of Medicine, IOM 7, 103, 108, 128, 180, 188, 195, 199
Intensivists 27, 38, 50
International Classification of Diseases, ICD, ICD-9, ICD-10 46, 47, 154, 155, 156, 195, 199, 201
Internist 50, 51, 79, 80, 99, 105, 184, 185
Interpersonal and Communication Skills 18, 37, 55, 71, 112

K
Kaiser Permanente 160

L
Length of Stay, LOS 19, 22, 34, 36, 43, 44, 48, 49, 52, 55, 71, 99, 191

M
Mayo Clinic 5, 138
Medical Knowledge 18, 19, 56, 72, 113, 121, 125, 126, 127, 131, 134, 135

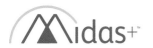

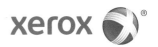

Manage, Measure, Monitor and Improve Care Delivery

With more than 2,000 clients, **Midas+ Solutions, a Xerox Company** is the preferred healthcare quality outcomes improvement and strategic performance management partner.

By leveraging our more than twenty-seven years of market domain expertise, Midas+ clients outperform the median national hospital quality scores for value-based purchasing and other pay-for-performance programs.

Midas+ Today

Market-leading provider of Care Performance solutions and services to optimize clinical and financial outcomes

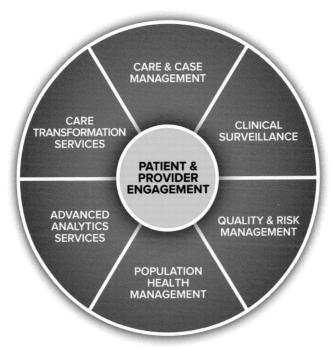

To learn more about Midas+, please visit
www.midasplus.com or contact us at **800.737.8835**

PRINTED IN THE UNITED STATES

9 780984 205134